Focus on Cancer

Springer

London
Berlin
Heidelberg
New York
Barcelona
Budapest
Hong Kong
Milan
Paris
Santa Clara
Singapore
Tokyo

Jocelyn Chamberlain and Sue Moss (Eds.)

Evaluation of Cancer Screening

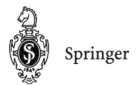 Springer

Jocelyn Chamberlain
Sue Moss

Cancer Screening Evaluation Unit, Section of Epidemiology
Institute of Cancer Research, Block D, Cotswold Road
Sutton, Surrey SM2 5NG, UK

ISBN 3-540-19957-8 Springer-Verlag Berlin Heidelberg New York

British Library Cataloguing in Publication Data
Evaluation of Cancer Screening. - (Focus on Cancer Series)
  I. Chamberlain, Jocelyn   II. Moss, Susan   III. Series
  616.994075
  ISBN   3-540-19957-8

Library of Congress Cataloging-in-Publication Data
Evaluation of Cancer Screening / Jocelyn Chamberlain and Sue Moss (eds.)
       p.   cm. -- (Focus on cancer)
  Includes bibliographical references and index.
  ISBN   3-540-19957-8 (pbk. : alk. paper)
  1. Cancer--Diagnosis--Evaluation.   2. Medical screening--Evaluation
  I. Chamberlain, Jocelyn, 1932-   . II. Moss, Sue, 1952-   . III. Series
  [DNLM: 1. Neoplasms--prevention & control.   2. Mass screening.
  3. Program Evaluation.   QZ 200 E913 1995]
  RA645.C3E975   1995
  362.1'96994--dc20
  DNLM/DLC
  for Library of Congress   95-23890

© Springer-Verlag London Limited 1996
Printed in Great Britain

Typeset by Richard Powell Editorial and Production Services, Basingstoke, Hants RG22 4TX
Printed and bound at the Athenæum Press Ltd., Gateshead, Tyne and Wear
28/3830-543210 Printed on acid-free paper

Contents

Series Editor's Foreword

Cancer is a major issue in the provision of health care. It is estimated that one in four people in developed countries are likely to develop it at some time. As longevity steadily increases, the incidence of malignant disease is expected to rise further. Important advances in the control of cancer have taken place and curative treatment has improved, notably in some of the rarer tumours, particularly in children. Advances in the more common cancers have been less marked, although adjunctive systemic treatment and population screening are lowering mortality from the most prevalent cancer – carcinoma of the breast. Despite this progress, complete control of malignant disease is still a long way off. However, our understanding of the molecular biology of cancer has increased enormously in recent years and the application of this knowledge holds considerable promise for developing new therapeutic strategies. As for prevention, the cause of most cancers is still poorly understood although it is clear that tobacco avoidance would prevent most lung cancers and several others.

Cancer is studied at many different levels: molecular and cellular biology, pathology in patients (particularly clinical trials), and prevention and populations (epidemiology). The psychosocial problems caused to patients and their families are being increasingly recognised and subjected to systematic study. Workers in the field, therefore, range from basic scientists to epidemiologists, from hospital specialists to community support teams. Each needs to have at least some knowledge of the role the others play. However, to bring all together in a single educational forum is impractical. Nevertheless, this ideal underlies the ethos of this series. Cancer issues are well served by a burgeoning literature of learned journals, newsletters, student textbooks and specialised monographs. Less available are concise overviews of general aspects for the busy oncologist and equally to those many professionals who are involved in the subject but are not specialists in it. Springer-Verlag's Focus on Cancer series has been designed to meet this information need. Each issue is devoted to a well-defined theme such as basic science and clinical application, diagnostic methods (including clinical appraisal of new technology), treatment, complications of cancer and psychosocial problems. The reader will judge whether this aim has been achieved and I will be pleased to receive comments and suggestions, including further topics for coverage in this series.

April, 1995   R. D. Rubens
United Medical and Dental Schools
Guy's and St Thomas's Hospitals, London

Preface

In the absence of effective primary prevention of cancer, "secondary prevention" by means of screening is, on the face of it, an attractive proposition for many cancer sites. Nevertheless, only for breast and cervical cancer is the benefit of screening considered sufficiently proven in many countries for a public-health population-based screening programme to be implemented.

As with other public-health interventions, there is a particular ethical responsibility on those providing screening to ensure that the chance of a person benefiting from it exceeds the chance of his being harmed by it. Therefore it is necessary to establish by research the extent of benefit, e.g. the proportion of deaths avoided or life-years gained, and to balance this against the disadvantages incurred through factors such as false-positive test results, overdiagnosis of non-progressive disease and opportunity costs of using public or private resources for this purpose.

The aim of this volume is to provide an up-to-date review of current evidence on the value of cancer screening. Following an initial chapter which outlines the general principles of screening and the research methodology required, individual chapters describe research-based evidence on the pros and cons of screening for ten different cancers. For each one, the size of the problem in terms of incidence and mortality is described and its aetiology is briefly reviewed, so as to indicate not only the feasibility of primary prevention, but also the high-risk groups at which screening might be targeted. Such evidence as there is on natural history is described, with an indication of how this could theoretically be altered by early detection. Estimates of the sensitivity and specificity of potential screening tests are summarised, and the findings of studies aimed at measuring reductions in mortality or incidence are reported. Evidence, which is usually sparse, on the side-effects and costs of screening is also summarised.

The two final chapters deal with psychological and economic aspects of screening, with an emphasis on the difficult methodological problems that measurement of these aspects entails.

It is hoped that this book will be of value to all health professionals with an interest in screening and cancer control, but especially to purchasers of health care, whether in the public or the private sector.

Sutton, 1995   JC
                                                                                   SM

The Editors and the Contributors

Dr Jackie Brown
Institute of Cancer Research, Section of Epidemiology
D Block, Cotswold Road, Sutton, Surrey SM2 5NG

Professor Jocelyn Chamberlain
Institute of Cancer Research, Section of Epidemiology
D Block, Cotswold Road, Sutton, Surrey SM2 5NG

Professor Howard Cuckle
Institute of Epidemiology and Health Services Research
Department of Clinical Medicine, The University of Leeds
34 Hyde Terrace, Leeds LS2 9LN

Dr Ruth Ellman
Institute of Cancer Research, Section of Epidemiology,
D Block, Cotswold Road, Sutton, Surrey SM2 5NG

Dr Jane Melia
Institute of Cancer Research, Section of Epidemiology
D Block, Cotswold Road, Sutton, Surrey SM2 5NG

Dr Sue Moss
Institute of Cancer Research, Section of Epidemiology
D Block, Cotswold Road, Sutton, Surrey SM2 5NG

1 – General Principles of Cancer Screening

Sue Moss

Introduction

Screening for cancer is based on the premise that earlier diagnosis of the disease, either in a precancerous state or at an earlier stage than that at which clinical presentation would otherwise take place, leads to a reduction in risk of mortality or development of invasive disease. Although the concept has been in existence for some time, only two sites, breast and cervix, have established screening programmes in the UK, although elsewhere, notably in the United States, screening for other sites, such as cancer of the prostate [14] is widely carried out.

Definition of Screening

This volume is in general concerned with population screening; that is the application of a test to an asymptomatic population in order to identify those subjects likely to have the disease in question.

There has been some debate about the difference between screening and case-finding; the latter term really applies to situations in which the subject who is tested presents to a physician with some complaint, not necessarily related to the disease which is tested for [22]. However, in some instances a subject will attend a physician in order to obtain a medical check-up or a specific screening test, and this would then fall into the category of screening [15].

Another situation which is discussed here but does not strictly fall into the definition of screening given above, is that in which a health education programme is used to promote the earlier detection of disease within a population either by increased awareness or by "self-screening" such as breast self-examination. Many of the evaluation measures described below are difficult to apply to such programmes; this is discussed in more detail later in this chapter.

Consideration of a Potential Screening Test

In considering the evaluation of a potential screening test for a given disease, the first decision must be whether the disease itself is a suitable candidate for screening. In general it should be a common health problem. However, some of the cancer sites now under consideration for screening have a comparatively low incidence. What is important is the cost of the screening test in relation to the potential yield of cancers (and eventually the life-years saved). This will also be affected by the number of times a screening test will need to be carried out. For example, if an effective screening test were developed for neuroblastoma it might only be necessary to screen each child once in order to detect the majority of cases at a curable stage. Similarly, a screening regime for colorectal cancer has been proposed which would involve a single screen by flexible sigmoidoscopy at age 50 or 55 [3]. In general, infrequent screening will be feasible for a disease which either occurs in a restricted age range, or which has a very long detectable preclinical phase.

Another possibility which may reduce the cost of screening for one disease is that of multiphasic screening, where screening tests for a number of diseases are carried out at the same time. This might be useful if established screening programmes such as that for breast cancer could be added to, a proposal currently being tested in the UK for ovarian cancer screening.

Some knowledge of the natural history of a disease is also essential for it to be suitable for screening. However, such knowledge can be difficult to obtain, and often it is data from screening studies themselves which provide the best information on natural history. The identification of a treatable, preclinical phase is essential before screening is considered. However, it is not always known which of the cases detected in this preclinical phase would progress to clinical disease if the natural history were not interrupted by screening. In the absence of such knowledge some overtreatment of non-progressive disease becomes inevitable. The implications of this are clearly more serious the more invasive the possible treatment, and for example it has been suggested that screening for prostate cancer should not yet even be evaluated in a randomised controlled trial for this reason [1].

There must also be an established treatment for the disease which is detected by screening together with some evidence that treatment at an earlier stage is associated with improved survival (over and above the "lead-time" discussed below). For screening tests which aim to detect a precancerous state, treatment of such a state is usually successful, although the possibility that treated subjects will remain at subsequent increased risk of the disease must be considered. For screening tests which are intended to detect cancer at an early stage, the aim is to detect cancer at a point before it has metastasised, and failure to advance diagnosis enough to achieve this may explain the ineffectiveness of some screening tests, such as screening by chest X-ray for lung cancer [11].

The evaluation of a screening programme can be seen as a series of phases, with the first phase being the development of the screening test itself. This will involve establishing that the test does in fact detect precursors of the disease, or early stage asymptomatic disease as appropriate. Examples of this are the recognition that levels of prostate specific antigen (PSA) are raised in men with asymptomatic prostate cancer, and the finding that certain types of human papilloma virus (HPV) are associated with cervical intraepithelial neoplasia (CIN) III. It will include developing satisfactory procedures and cut-off levels for measuring or reading the screening test in order to decide which cases needed further investigation. Another requisite is that there is a diagnostic procedure which will determine precisely which of those cases found positive by the screening test truly do have the disease in question.

Evaluating the Performance of a Test

The second phase will then involve estimating the acceptability, sensitivity, specificity, and yield of the screening test. Satisfactory levels of each of these are necessary, although not sufficient, conditions for the success of any screening programme.

Acceptability

The uptake of screening is crucial to the eventual success of any screening programme, and any proposed screening test needs to be acceptable to the population at which it is aimed. This phase of the evaluation of screening may therefore include some assessment of various methods of improving compliance, for example by the use of personal invitations and specified appointments, experimenting with different wording of letters, and the provision of different types and levels of background information about the test. Some "selection bias" may often be present, with those subjects who accept the offer of a screening test being at either higher or lower risk of the disease than the general population. Although such bias can also affect the eventual success of a programme, it may be difficult to quantify at this stage of evaluation where there will not in general be a control population. It is also possible that the non-attenders may be at similar risk of incidence of the disease, but will be those subjects who tend to present at a later stage, and so will be at increased risk of dying from the disease. Such a bias was observed in the UK Trial of Early Detection of Breast Cancer [28].

It is also important that the follow-up diagnostic procedures to be carried out on those subjects found positive by the initial screening test are acceptable. There will inevitably be some false positive cases from the initial screening test, and unpleasant diagnostic procedures in these may lead to a reduction in subsequent compliance with screening.

Sensitivity

The sensitivity of a screening test is the ability of the test to detect true cases of the disease. In the past, this has often been estimated by counting as "true positives" the screen-detected cases plus those cases occurring in a set period (often 12 months) following a negative screen, usually called "interval cases". The sensitivity of the test is then calculated as the proportion of these positives which were detected by the screening test [5]. It is now recognised that this can produce a biased estimate of sensitivity, due to the fact that not all the "interval" cases would have been present or detectable at the time of the screening test, and also that some of the cases detected by screening would not otherwise have presented during the "follow-up" period considered, and some might never have presented clinically at all. An alternative method of estimating sensitivity has been proposed [7] which is now more often used in the evaluation of screening trials or established programmes. This "proportional incidence" method, which was used to estimate sensitivity in the analysis of the Swedish two-counties breast screening trial [26], looks at the proportion of the estimated incidence of disease which would have occurred in the absence of screening, whose diagnosis has been advanced by the screening test.

This is done by calculating the incidence of interval cancers in a given period following a negative screen, expressed as a proportion of the underlying incidence in the attenders for screening. The latter requires an estimate of the incidence in a comparable population and also that in non-attenders for screening in order to adjust for any selection bias. Such data may not always be readily available for the initial evaluation of a screening test, but will be provided by a randomised trial, in which a defined population is randomly allocated to a group offered screening or to an unscreened control group. For example, if interval cancers make up 20% of the expected incidence in a given time period after screening, it is assumed that screening has advanced the diagnosis of the remaining 80%.

Specificity

The specificity of a screening test is the ability to identify true negatives correctly. Since the false positives of screening will be identified by the subsequent diagnostic procedure, specificity can be calculated as the proportion of all true negatives (screened negatives plus false positives) correctly classified as negative by the screening test. The importance of achieving high specificity depends to some extent on the cost of the follow-up diagnostic procedures, and on how invasive these procedures are, but among these costs must be included the anxiety which will almost inevitably be caused in a healthy person who is wrongly labelled as "positive" for even a short period of time. For the majority of screening tests, there is a trade-off between sensitivity and specificity. For example, if the percentage of all true cases which are identified as positive by a test falls with an increasing level of some test measurement, then increasing the cut-off point for the screening test will increase the specificity, as fewer cases will be wrongly selected for further investigation, but will decrease the sensitivity as more truly positive cases will be missed. However, using a combination of screening tests can increase both the sensitivity and specificity compared with those of a single test. For example, the use of two-view mammography as compared with a single view can both increase the sensitivity of screening (since some cases will be detected on the second view that were missed on the first) and increase the specificity (since some suspicious lesions which would have been recalled on one-view alone are sufficiently clear on the second view to remove suspicion).

Yield of Cancer Detected

The yield of a screening test, particularly that in previously unscreened subjects, is clearly crucial, and this will depend on the underlying level of the disease in the population. It is often expressed as a "prevalence to incidence ratio", that is, the number of cases found per 1000 population screened for the first time compared with the expected number of cases arising each year per 1000 people in a control population. However, this will be affected both by the sensitivity of the screening test and by the duration of the preclinical detectable phase of the disease.

Assuming 100% sensitivity, these are related by the equation $P = mI$ where P is the prevalence of preclinical disease, I is the underlying incidence rate and m is the mean duration of the preclinical detectable phase [34].

Another measure used is the positive predictive value of the screening test, which is the probability that a subject found positive by the test will in fact have the disease in question. The advantage of this measure is that it is largely dependent on the specificity of the test and the underlying prevalence of disease in the population.

Evaluating the Effectiveness of Screening

Randomised Controlled Trials

A randomised controlled trial is the most definitive method of evaluating the effectiveness of screening. If estimates from the early phase of evaluation were satisfactory, then the next phase could be the implementation of large-scale ran-domised trials. In practice, early studies are often designed so that they can be ex-panded into larger randomised trials if successful. Such randomised trials generally need to involve large numbers of subjects due to relatively low levels of disease, and will often, therefore, need to be multicentre and/or take place in more than one country. They should be designed to have the power to detect useful reductions in mortality (or in incidence of invasive disease if this is the aim of the screening test) at a level which would be considered important by health planners. A point sometimes overlooked is that cases diagnosed before the start of a screening trial cannot benefit from that screening. When calculating the sample size required for a screening trial, the estimate of mortality from the disease in an initially disease-free control group should, therefore, exclude the mortality due to such cases, and possible methods of such estimation have been proposed.

Moss et al. [19] describe a method, originally applied to a trial of screening for colorectal cancer, in which year by year survival rates are applied to disease incidence rates for the appropriate age–sex distribution of population being considered, to obtain an estimate of the number of deaths in successive years after the start of a trial. Straatman and Verbeek [25] present a "shortcut" method, which, however, assumes incidence and mortality rates to be constant over time.

In general, randomised trials are analysed by looking at the disease-specific mortality, using the total number of subjects in each group as the denominator, and employing a Poisson test statistic. Analyses based on case-fatality rates are liable to be biased due to the potential of screening to detect slower-growing or non-progressive disease. However, it has been argued that once the number of cases in the study and control groups have become equal, then an unbiased analysis is possible based on mortality using these cases as the denominator. The advantage is that such an analysis is more powerful; for example, a significant reduction in breast cancer mortality has been demonstrated using the method in women aged 40–49 years at entry to the Health Insurance Plan (HIP) breast screening study [6], whereas previous analyses had failed to show a significant reduction.

It should perhaps be noted that screening tests designed to reduce disease-specific mortality cannot be expected to have a significant impact on all-cause mortality, although the lack of evidence of such an impact has been used to justify claims for the ineffectiveness of screening [24].

The reduction in risk of disease-specific death found in prospective population-based trials, although useful for public health planning, is an underestimate of the size of effect in screened people, since such trials must necessarily include deaths in people who did not attend for screening. With knowledge of the proportion of non-attenders an estimate of the reduction in risk in screened people can be made. For example, a relative risk of 0.70 in a population, of whom 25% did not attend for screening, translates to a relative risk of 0.60 in screened people, assuming that the underlying risk in screened and unscreened subjects is the same. If the underlying risk of death in non-attenders is greater (selection bias) the reduction in risk in screened people will be greater [31].

In the evaluation of a screening trial, completeness of data collection is essential. In particular, efforts must be made to ensure that the identification of cases and deaths is as accurate in the control population, and in the study population where cases are not detected by screening, as for the screen-detected cases.

If a population-based screening programme is to be introduced, it should ideally be demonstrated that the programme is cost-effective in comparison with other health promotion or intervention policies. This is generally done by comparing the financial costs of screening with the estimated "life-years saved". Financial costs will include not only the costs of the screening programme, but those of the follow-up test, and of early treatment as opposed to late.

However, in weighing up all the potential costs and benefits there are other, non-financial aspects which must be considered. There may be potential harmful effects of the screening test, such as the possible carcinogenic effects of radiation in mammography. By detecting (and treating) cases early, screening will increase the length of time for which patients know they have the disease, and possibly diagnose some cases which would otherwise have remained undiscovered, and this will increase morbidity to some extent. There is also the possibility that subjects screened negative will be given false reassurance, which may lead them subsequently to ignore symptoms and present with the disease at a later stage than they would have done otherwise. There are also possible psychological costs to be considered, such as increases in both short- and long-term anxiety in those invited for screening, and particularly in those found positive by the initial screening test.

On the benefit side, there may be not only a reduction in mortality, but improved quality of life due to earlier treatment, for example from the treatment of breast cancer by wide local excision as opposed to mastectomy. Other potential benefits of screening may include an increased health awareness among individuals as a result of their attendance for screening, and reassurance for those found negative that they are free of the disease.

Implementation of Population Screening Programmes

The final phase of the evaluation will be the implementation of population-based screening. It is now recognised that such programmes still need careful monitoring and evaluation, since the real-life setting may differ from the rigorously controlled procedures of a randomised trial. Again, it will be a long time before such programmes demonstrate an effect on mortality, and this effect may be difficult to measure for reasons similar to those affecting non-randomised trials, so that evaluation and interim measures of yield, acceptability and coverage and of sensitivity (by the monitoring of interval cases) will be essential [8].

Alternative Methods of Evaluation

The need for randomised trials with mortality as an end-point, at least for previously unproven screening tests, is because of a number of biases which affect other comparisons. Comparison of the survival of screen-detected with other cases is hampered by lead-time bias, and length bias [34]. Lead-time bias [10] arises because screening will detect cases at an earlier point in time than that at which they would otherwise have been diagnosed. This results in longer survival from diagnosis to death, even if death occurs at the same time as it would in the absence of screening. Length-bias arises due to the tendency of screening to detect slow-growing cases which spend longer in the preclinical detectable phase. Such cases may tend to be associated with improved prognosis compared with fast-growing cases which are more likely to present during the intervals between screening. Selection bias, already described above, affects comparisons of attenders and non-attenders for screening, and is a particular problem in case-control studies (discussed below).

However, although the randomised controlled trial is the ideal means by which a potential screening policy should be evaluated, this will not always be feasible. For example, cervical screening became widespread before it had been rigorously evaluated, by which time it would have been ethically impossible to implement a randomised controlled trial. In some situations there may be constraints preventing individual randomisation, for example it may not be feasible to introduce screening without contamination of the control group. Randomisation of geographical units or clusters is possible, but if these are large this can result in bias [2]. If a randomised trial is not feasible, a controlled comparison of geographical districts is a possibility, but again evaluation can be difficult if external factors are not allowed for. These include not only differences in the underlying incidence and/or mortality in the different districts, but also possible different treatment policies which may affect outcome. Such differences have hampered evaluation of the UK Trial of Early Detection of Breast Cancer, in which different interventions took place in two pairs of districts, with a further four districts providing a comparison population [27].

When only a largely retrospective analysis is possible, most attempts at evaluation of screening programmes use geographical comparisons of different regions or countries, and/or analysis of trends over time. The main problem with such analyses is in determining what the underlying trends in incidence and/or mortality were before the introduction of screening, and thus in determining how much of any reduction is due to the screening programme and how much to extraneous factors. In such situations, it is often also difficult to establish the frequency or coverage of screening which has produced any benefit.

Use of Surrogate Outcome Measures

Recently, the possible use of surrogate outcome measures has been proposed as a means of both reducing the size of randomised trial needed to evaluate screening tests, and of obtaining an answer from such trials earlier than is the case if they use mortality as an end-point. The idea is that instead of following subjects through to death (or invasive disease), an interim measure be used from which eventual mortality can be predicted. Such a proposal has so far been made specifically for breast cancer, with size, nodal status and grade being used as surrogate outcome measures from which eventual mortality can be estimated [9].

The use of such measures is still largely experimental and is mainly valid in situations where the effectiveness of a screening test is proven in one situation, and a variation is being tested. For example, their use is planned to evaluate a trial of breast screening in the UK in which the effectiveness of 1-yearly and 3-yearly mammography is being compared. It should be noted that the power of a trial for a given sample size is only increased if it is assumed that there is no error in the prediction of mortality from the surrogate measures. This is a strong assumption, particularly where data from one country are being used to predict mortality in another.

Morrison [17] has identified a number of factors which may affect the accuracy with which analysis of surrogate outcome measures will predict mortality, the majority tending to result in an underestimate of the effect of screening. These include the fact that even within a given level of some prognostic factor, there will be cases with and without undetected metastases, so that screening will be of benefit even within this level. If fairly broad measurement categories are used, the prognosis may vary within these categories (e.g. number of involved nodes within "node positive cases"). There may also be measurement error, both in screen-detected and other cases, but with a tendency also to less complete data being available for non screen-detected cases. There is also the possibility that non-progressive cases detected by screening may not be correctly identified. Finally, the prediction may be affected by treatment differences – either a correlation of the effect of treatment with stage and mode of detection, or changes in the effectiveness of treatment with time over the duration of a trial. By using data on stage from the HIP breast screening trial as surrogate outcome measures, Morrison found that the predicted difference in mortality between the study and control groups was considerably less than that observed.

Case-Control Studies of Screening

Case-control studies have been widely used to evaluate screening in situations where there are no population controls. In a randomised controlled trial, the risk of death from the disease in the population offered screening is estimated relative to that in the control population. Case-control studies of screening generally estimate the odds of becoming a "case" in subjects who are or are not screened, and thus estimate the relative risk in acceptors of screening compared with non-acceptors. As discussed above such comparisons are liable to be affected by selection bias. For example, a case-control study carried out within one of the screening centres of the UK Trial of Early Detection of Breast Cancer [20], which had an overall 20% reduction in breast cancer mortality relative to the comparison districts, found a risk of 0.5 in the acceptors relative to the non-acceptors. This suggests that the non-acceptors were at higher risk of mortality than the comparison population. Some case-control studies have attempted to adjust for factors associated with compliance in order to reduce the effect of selection bias, but the effect of such adjustment in estimates of risk leaves some doubt that all selection bias has been removed [18]. The selection of both cases [16] and controls [33] in these studies is crucial in ensuring the relative risk is correctly estimated.

Two types of case-control study have been identified, according to whether the screening test is designed to detect precursors of the disease, or an early stage of the disease itself [23]. In the first instance, "cases" will be cases of invasive disease since this is what the screening test is aiming to prevent; any such cases detected by screening need separate consideration since their screening history will differ from that of symptomatic cases [12]. Controls should be alive and free of the disease at the time of diagnosis of the case, and the screening history of both cases and controls measured up to the time of diagnosis of the cases. For cases detected by screening, that screening test should *not* be included in the history; moreover, controls for such a case should have been screened at the same time as the case (and again that screen excluded from the screening history).

In the second type of study, where the aim of screening is to detect early stage disease, cases should be deaths from the disease, and the screening history of the case should include any screening test which led to detection of the case. Controls should be alive at the time of death of the case, and again should be free of the disease at the time of diagnosis of the case, in order that they have had the same opportunity for screening in the relevant time period [23].

Mathematical Models of Screening

Data from screening trials and studies often provide information which can be used to develop mathematical models of disease natural histories. Such models are useful not only in providing further insight into the natural history, but also in extrapolating from the results of a particular screening trial or protocol to a programme with a different screening interval, or different ages at which screening is to be offered.

The simplest models are macrosimulation models, which represent the disease natural history as a series of states, and apply transition rates between these states to cohorts of people [13]. However, such models are relatively inflexible compared with "microsimulation" models, which apply transitions to individual subjects. Such models have been developed and applied for both breast and cervical cancer screening [30, 29, 21].

Mathematical models, such as that developed by Walter and Day [32], which assume that the preclinical disease phase has a given distribution, and then use data from screening studies to estimate the parameters for the distribution, are useful in providing estimates of lead-time, again with implications for frequency of screening. Such models become more complex for diseases with a precancerous state as well as an asymptomatic invasive phase [4].

Selection of High-Risk Groups for Screening

Targeting screening at those subgroups of the population at highest risk will increase its cost-effectiveness, since the yield of cancers detected per screen will be greater. However, with the exception of selection by age it is difficult in general to identify sufficiently large subgroups with high enough increased risk for screening to have a significant impact on the rates of disease in the general population. Screening may, however, be justified as cost-effective in such subgroups where it is not in the general population, e.g. in an occupationally exposed group, or in those with a strong family history. However, it should be borne in mind that screening needs to be established as effective before there are grounds for implementing it even in a high-risk group.

Promotion of Early Diagnosis

Some measures aimed at the early detection of cancer are not truly "screening" as defined above, but merit consideration here. The difference is that they are largely health promotion ventures, and it is usually the effect of the education intervention (and sometimes provision of easier referral facilities) that is being measured or evaluated, rather than the test or examination itself. Programmes which fall into this category include the promotion of breast self-examination, and encouragement of awareness about changes in moles to leads to earlier diagnosis of melanoma. In particular, sensitivity and specificity have little meaning in such a context. It is essential that such programmes be followed through to the same end-points of incidence or mortality as randomised trials of screening. However, in such situations identification of a suitable control population for comparison is difficult because any publicity will affect all subjects in the area, so that it is usually necessary to use either geographic comparisons and/or comparisons of time trends. Selection bias is again a particular problem if comparing cases found or not found as a result of education, and lead time and length bias will have the same effect as before.

Ethical Issues

There is a growing awareness of the ethical issues surrounding screening. It has long been recognised that screening has a unique rôle among medical interventions, in that the screening is offered to healthy subjects. There is, therefore, a strong responsibility to provide full information to the subject and to treat any screening detected abnormalities quickly. (The situation is somewhat akin to immunisation, but whereas the whole community benefits from mass immunisation, the only people to benefit directly from mass screening are those subjects who have disease diagnosed by screening and whose death is delayed as a result.)

It is essential that subjects being offered a screening test are given all possible information. Obviously if the test is being offered as part of a trial (randomised or otherwise) this should be clearly stated. It should be made clear that screening is not 100% sensitive, i.e. that being screened negative does not mean that the subject is either definitely free of the disease or will not develop it in the future. This will avoid false reassurance which might lead to the subject subsequently ignoring symptoms and presenting later than otherwise due to screening. It may also be important in some places to avoid legal action if a screened negative subject subsequently develops cancer. The provision of information on early symptoms of disease may lead to an enhancement of the effectiveness of the screening programme; for example the promotion of "breast awareness" by a breast screening programme may lead to a shift in stage at diagnosis over and above that due to screening.

Genetic Issues

It has long been known that some cancers are at least in part hereditary, and that subjects with one or more affected first degree relative will be at greater risk of developing the disease themselves. A growing number of clinics exist to counsel such subjects, but how they should be treated with respect to screening is not always clear. Although they are at increased risk, there is usually no reason to believe that an unproven screening test should be effective in such subjects, yet it is seldom believed ethical to allow them to be entered into a randomised trial, and they are commonly offered screening.

The identification of cancer genes opens up a whole new potential field of cancer screening. If the identification of a subject carrying such a gene is considered as a screening test in itself, however, it should be evaluated as rigorously as any other test. The treatment to be offered to such subjects is of particular concern, since it is likely that at least some subjects who will not develop the disease will be treated, yet the risk is so high that radical treatment may be considered. Although the gene may be identified, the natural history in terms of when cancer may develop may not be known. The psychological consequences of carrying out such a screening test also merit serious consideration, particularly if no immediate treatment is to be offered.

References

1. Adami H, Baron J, Rothman K (1994) Ethics of a prostate cancer screening trial. Lancet 343:958–960.

2. Alexander F, Roberts MM, Lutz W, Hepburn W (1989) Randomisation by cluster and the problem of social class bias. J Epidemiol Community Health 43:29–36.

3. Atkin WS, Cuzick J, Northover JMA, Whynes DK (1993) Prevention of colorectal cancer by once-only sigmoidoscopy. Lancet 341:736–340.

4. Brookmeyer R, Day NE (1987) Two-stage models of the analysis of cancer screening data. Biometrics 43:657–669.

5. Chamberlain J, Rogers P, Price JL, Ginks S, Nathan BE, Burn I (1975) Validity of clinical examination and mammography as screening tests for breast cancer. Lancet ii:1026–1037.

6. Chu KC, Smart CR, Tarone RE (1988) Analysis of breast cancer mortality and stage distribution by age for the Health Insurance Plan clinical trial. J Natl Cancer Inst 80:1125–1132.

7. Day NE (1985) Estimating the sensitivity of a screening test. J Epidemiol Community Health 39:364–366.

8. Day NE, Williams DR, Khaw KT (1989) Breast cancer screening programmes. The development of a monitoring and evaluation system. Br J Cancer 59:954–958.

9. Day NE (1991) Surrogate measures in the design of breast screening trials. In: Miller AB, Chamberlain J, Day NE, Hakama M, Prorok PC (eds) Cancer screening. UICC project on evaluation of screening for cancer. Cambridge University Press, Cambridge, pp 391–403.

10. Feinleib M, Zelen M (1969) Some pitfalls in the evaluation of screening programs. Arch Environ Health 19:412–415.

11. Fontana RS, Sanderson DR, Woolner LB, Taylor WF, Miller WE, Muhm JR (1986) Lung cancer screening. The Mayo program. J Occup Med 28:746–750.

12. IARC Working Group on Evaluation of Cervical Cancer Screening Programmes (1986) Screening for squamous cervical cancer: duration of low risk after negative results of cervical cytology and its implication for screening policies. Br Med J 293:659–664.

13. Knox EG (1973) A simulation system for screening procedures. In: McLachlan G (ed) The future and present indicatives (Problems and Progress in Medical Care IX). Nuffield Provincial Hospitals Trust, Oxford, pp 19–30.

14. Lu-Yao GL, Greenberg ER (1994) Changes in prostate cancer incidence and treatment in USA. Lancet 343:251–254.

15. Miller AB (1985) Principles of screening and the evaluation of screening programs. In: Miller AB (ed) Screening for cancer. Academic Press, Orlando, pp 3–24.

16. Morrison AS (1982) Case definition in case-control studies of the efficacy of screening. Am J Epidemiol 115:6–8.

17. Morrison AS (1991) Intermediate determinants of mortality in the definition of screening. Int J Epidemiol 20:642–650.

18. Moss SM (1991) Case-control studies of screening. Int J Epidemiol 20(1):1–6.

19. Moss SM, Draper GJ, Hardcastle JD, Chamberlain J (1987) Calculation of sample size in trials for early diagnosis of disease. Int J Epidemiol 16:104–110.

20. Moss SM, Summerley ME, Thomas BT, Ellman R, Chamberlain JOP (1992) A case-control evaluation of the effect of breast cancer screening in the United Kingdom trial of early detection of breast cancer. J Epidemiol Community Health 46:362–364.

21. Parkin DM, Moss SM (1986) An evaluation of screening policies for cervical cancer in England and Wales using a computer simulation model. J Epidemiol Community Health 40:143–153.

22. Sackett DL, Holland WW (1875) Controversy in the detection of disease. Lancet ii:357–359.

23. Sasco AJ, Day NE, Walter SD (1986) Case-control studies for the evaluation of screening. J Chronic Dis 39:399–405.
24. Skrabanek P (1985) False premises and false promises of breast cancer screening. Lancet ii:316–319.
25. Straatman H, Verbeek A (1990) Shortcut method to calculate the sample size in trials of screening for chronic disease. J Clin Epidemiol 43:1261–1266.
26. Tabar L, Fagerberg G, Day NE, Holmberg L (1987) What is the optimum interval between mammographic screening examinations? Br J Cancer 55:547–551.
27. UK Trial of Early Detection of Breast Cancer Group (1981) Trial of early detection of breast cancer: description of method. Br J Cancer 44:618–627.
28. UK Trial of Early Detection of Breast Cancer Group (1988) First results on mortality reduction in the UK Trial of Early Detection of Breast Cancer. Lancet ii:411–416.
29. van Ballegooijen M, Habbema JDF, van Oortmarssen GJ, Koopmanschap MA, Lubbe JTN, van Agt HME (1992) Preventive pap-smears: balancing costs, risks and benefits. Br J Cancer 65:930–933.
30. van Ineveld BM, van Oortmarssen GJ, de Koning HJ, Boer R, van der Maas PJ (1993) How cost-effective is breast cancer screening in different EC countries? Eur J Cancer 29A(12):1663–1668.
31. Wald NJ, Chamberlain J, Hackshaw J (1993) A Report of the European Society for Mastology Breast Cancer Screening Evaluation Committee. Breast 2:209–216.
32. Walter SD, Day NE (1983) Estimation of the duration of a preclinical disease state using screening data. Am J Epidemiol 118:865–886.
33. Weiss NS (1983) Control definition in case-control studies of the efficacy of screening and diagnostic testing. Am J Epidemiol 118:457–460.
34. Zelen M, Feinleib M (1969) On the theory of screening for chronic diseases. Biometrika 56:601–614.

2 – Screening for Cancer of the Cervix

Sue Moss

Introduction

Cervical cancer is the fifth most common cancer in the world, with over 400 000 new cases reported each year [81]. It is also one of the few cancers for which a screening test is available which is generally accepted as efficacious, despite the fact that it has never been evaluated by means of a randomised controlled trial. However, it is clear that although underlying trends in incidence make it difficult to estimate the effect of screening quantitatively, screening has so far failed to reduce the impact of the disease to the extent which might be thought feasible.

Epidemiology of Cervical Cancer

Cervical cancer is the most common cancer in women in developing countries, and the fourth most common in women in Europe and North America. Age-standardised incidence rates for 1985 were 9.9 per 100 000 in North America and 46.8 per 100 000 in Southern Africa [63]. In England and Wales in 1987 there were 3972 new cases registered, giving an age-standardised rate of 11.6 per 100 000 [59].

Age-standardised mortality rates for 1985 ranged between 3.6 per 100 000 in North America and 24.3 per 100 000 in Eastern Africa. Mortality rates are high in tropical South America and Central America, with age-standardised rates of 17.4 per 100 000 and 15.4 per 100 000, respectively. Rates in the European areas are between 3.8 and 5.1 per 100 000 with the exception of Eastern Europe, with an age-standardised rate of 8.8 per 100 000 [65]. There were 1647 deaths from cervical cancer in England and Wales in 1992, a rate of 3.9 per 100 000 age-standardised to the world population [59].

The five-year survival rates of US whites with cervical cancer have been estimated as 99.1% for carcinoma in situ, 92.2% for locally invasive disease, 49.2% for regionally invasive cancer and 3.1% for cases with distant metastases. Equivalent figures for US blacks were 99.1%, 80.5%, 40.5% and 3.4% respectively [34]. In England and Wales, the five-year relative survival for in situ cases is 99.2%, and for all invasive cases is nearly 60% [58].

Trends in both incidence and mortality in many countries have been affected by varying levels of screening, and, as discussed below, decreasing trends are frequently used as evidence of the effectiveness of screening. In certain countries where the mortality from cervical cancer has increased since the 1960s, this is probably ascribable to some extent to changes in coding practices of cause of death [22].

The incidence of cervical cancer is most common in women aged over 30 years. In some countries, such as the UK and Australia, there has been an increase in both incidence and mortality in young women in recent years, and it is likely that this is a "cohort effect", and that such women will remain at increased risk throughout their lifetime. There is now evidence from the United States that a similar increase is being observed there in women below age 50 years.

The strongest risk factor for cervical cancer is sexual behaviour, with an increased risk being associated with early age at first intercourse, a woman's number of sexual partners [9], and the number of partners which a woman's male partner has [10]. It now appears almost certain that a sexually transmitted agent, probably one or more specific types of human papilloma virus, has a causal role in the disease aetiology [70]. Use of oral contraceptives has also been found to be associated with an increased risk [80], even after adjustment for sexual behaviour as a confounding factor, although it has been suggested the risk may be confined to adenocarcinomas [11]. Cigarette smoking has also been implicated, and a possible mechanism has been proposed in which smoking results in local immunosuppression in the cervical epithelium [6]. Despite suggestions that certain nutrients such as carotenoids, vitamins A and C and folate may be associated with a decreased risk of cervical cancer, the role, if any, of diet is not clear [82].

The Natural History of Cervical Cancer

It is generally accepted that invasive cervical cancer is the final stage of a continuous disease process, in which dysplasia arises in a normal cervical epithelium, and progresses through carcinoma in situ to invasive cancer. Studies of the prevalence and incidence of the various stages of the disease have led to the conclusion that a percentage of cases of mild or moderate dysplasia will regress without any intervention. Coppleson and Brown [18] attempted to develop a model of natural history of the disease based on age specific prevalence rates of dysplasia and carcinoma in situ derived from screening studies and incidence rates of invasive carcinoma, making a variety of assumptions about the sensitivity of the screening test. They found that it was only possible to develop a satisfactory model by allowing a significant amount of regression from carcinoma in situ to dysplasia or normal. A later study from British Columbia, in which data from two age cohorts of women were used, also concluded that regression of both carcinoma in situ and dysplasia occurs, with the probability of carcinoma in situ progressing to invasive cancer increasing with age [8].

More recently an analysis of data from Toronto, during a period in which cases of lesser degrees of dysplasia were largely followed-up cytologically, has found that the risk of progressing to malignancy, as found in a subsequent smear, increased with increasing degree of dysplasia [56].

A number of simulation models of the natural history of cervical cancer have also been developed. The earliest such model was that developed by Knox [42], who estimated transition rates between various disease states for a cohort of women. More recent models have been more flexible, and have modelled the histories of individual women. Parkin [62] derived a range of natural histories, with the median duration of dysplasia ranging from 2.2 to 2.6 years, and the median duration of progressive carcinoma in situ from 6.5 to 12.2 years. Habbema et al. [35], using the MISCAN computer simulation program, estimated a total mean duration in the "non-invasive preclinical state" of progressive disease of 10 years.

The original classification of Pap smears as class I to V is now rarely used. Most cytologists now use the terms mild, moderate or severe dysplasia, or the terminology of mild, moderate or severe dyskaryosis which is recommended by the British Society for Clinical Cytology [27]. The terminology of cervical intraepithelial neoplasia (CIN) is used by histopathologists with progression from CIN1 through CIN2 to CIN3 or carcinoma in situ, but concerns about variability in reporting have led some to call for this to be replaced by a two-category classification [67].

The "Pap" Test

The Papanicolaou or "Pap" test was developed in the 1930s by George Papanicolaou, who had earlier observed malignant changes in vaginal smears taken from patients with cervical cancer [61]; a similar observation had also been made in Rumania by Dr Aurel Babes [5]. In the late 1940s it was realised both that sampling from the uterine cervix was more efficient than taking a vaginal smear, and that the presence of carcinoma in situ (i.e. cancerous changes confined to the epithelium) could also be identified in the samples, thus identifying the cervical smear as a potential screening test.

The technique now most widely used to prepare a Pap smear is the cervical scrape technique introduced by Ayre [4], which obtains cells from the squamocolumnar junction, or transitional zone, of the uterine cervix, in the region of which the majority of precursor lesions of invasive squamous carcinoma of the cervix arise.

In developed countries screening by "Pap" smears became steadily more widespread during the 1960s, and evidence of associated reductions in the incidence of invasive disease and in mortality increased confidence in its effectiveness. As a result, the test has never been rigorously evaluated by means of a randomised trial, since by the time the need for such evaluation was identified, screening was widely implemented in many countries, and generally considered so effective as to make it ethically impossible to carry out a trial in which a control group would be deprived of screening.

Evidence for the Effectiveness of Screening

The aim of screening for cervical cancer is to detect lesions in the precancerous state before the onset of invasive disease. Screening should, therefore, reduce not only mortality from cervical cancer but also the incidence of invasive cancer. However, screening will also pick up some cases of asymptomatic invasive cancer as well as in situ disease, so that incidence rates may not fall as rapidly as expected. Mortality is also a more reliable endpoint because reporting of death is liable to be more complete than that of cancer incidence.

Much of the current evidence for the effectiveness of cervical screening comes from studies of populations where organised screening programmes have been implemented, in which trends in the incidence of invasive cervical cancer and in mortality from the disease are compared either with those from the same geographical area before the introduction of screening, or with those from a similar nearby population with no organised screening programme.

The most convincing evidence comes from Scandinavia, where mass screening programmes were introduced at different times in different countries. In Finland, screening began in the mid-1960s and became nationwide in the early 1970s. At that time it was targeted at the age-group 30–55 years although it now covers women aged 25–60 years with a 5-year screening interval. There is a high coverage of between 70 and 80% although with a large percentage of smears also taken outside the organised programme. By 1980, the annual incidence of invasive disease had fallen by around 60%, with the greatest reduction apparent below age 50 [46]. The mortality rate also fell by 70% over a similar period, from 6.8 to 2.0 per 100 000, with a reduction of 80% at ages 30–59 years. There was a slight decreasing trend in the incidence in young women aged 30–39 before the introduction of screening. However, a comparison with the neighbouring country of Estonia, which has no mass screening programme, shows that whereas incidence and mortality rates have decreased in both countries since the mid-1960s, the decrease in Estonia has been far less pronounced than that in Finland [1].

In Iceland, a screening programme for all women aged 25–69 years was introduced in 1969, with screening starting some 5 years earlier in the capital. Incidence and mortality data are available from 1955, and examination of age-standardised rates shows both to have been increasing before the introduction of screening. Incidence fell markedly between 1969 and 1978, with a decrease of over 80% in women aged 40–59 years, although rates increased in women aged 20–29 years over this time period [71]. Mortality rates also fell over the period 1970 to 1980 [37], with an 80% decrease at ages 40–49 years, but an increase in the age group 25–29 years. In Sweden, screening began in counties in the south of the country in 1964, and the programme has been nationwide since 1977 when the city of Gothenborg began screening. The age-group invited for screening at first varied between counties, but since 1967 there have been national guidelines of 4-yearly screening between the ages of 30 and 49 years. However, as in Finland, it is estimated that a very high percentage of smears are taken outside the organised screening programme, although the guidelines have recently been revised to cover ages 20–59 years with a 3-yearly interval. The incidence of invasive cervical cancer fell steadily between 1965 and 1980, and analysis by year-of-birth cohorts showed steady decreases in age groups 35–59 years. Mortality also decreased markedly from 1960 onwards, with the decrease restricted to women below age 50 years [40].

In contrast, in Denmark and Norway only limited geographical areas were covered by organised screening programmes in the 1960s and 1970s, and the reductions in incidence and mortality were correspondingly smaller.

In Denmark, the decision to introduce organised screening programmes was left to individual counties, with no national guidelines. Between 1962 and 1980 nine counties introduced organised screening, covering approximately 40% of women, but sufficient smears were being taken in the country as a whole to cover the entire population. Between the late 1960s and 1980 both incidence and mortality from cervical cancer fell in Denmark as a whole, the incidence declining from 31.7 to 22.3 per 100 000. However, a study relating trends in incidence in different counties to the local authority smear-taking activity found the greatest decreases in areas with organised programmes with lower decreases in areas with no organised programmes but high screening activity, and only small reductions in those areas with low screening activity [49].

In Norway, only one area, Ostfold County, was involved in organised screening in a research project in which women aged 25–59 years were invited for five screening rounds between 1959 and 1977. Over the whole period, incidence was reduced by 22% and mortality by 17% compared with expected, but with greater decreases in the latter half of the study [64].

Since the late 1960s there have been a number of reports from the United States and from Canada of decreases in the incidence of invasive cervical cancer and in mortality from the disease associated with the introduction of cervical screening. The size of the decreases, and the fact that they are largely concentrated in the age-group most comprehensively screened, supports the hypothesis that the falls are due to screening, although the lack of comparison populations makes it difficult to draw firm conclusions, and there have been suggestions that mortality rates were also falling in areas less affected by screening [2]. However, an analysis which considered the intensity of screening in different areas of Canada concluded that the level of screening had a significant effect on the size of reduction in mortality from cervical cancer [51]. Similarly, a study in the United States found a positive correlation between level of screening in various states and the size of the decrease in mortality [21].

In Japan, a study comparing decreases in cervix cancer mortality over the period where screening became widespread found a significantly greater reduction in those areas with a high coverage rate of screening than in control areas only when the analysis was restricted to those areas with the highest initial mortality [43].

In the Netherlands, a 3-yearly screening programme was introduced in 1976, with screening starting in pilot regions, and offered to women aged 35–54 years [26]. In Nijmegen, one of the pilot areas, the incidence of invasive disease in women in this age group fell from 18.6 per 100 000 to 3.3 per 100 000 between 1970 and 1985. The mortality from cervical cancer in the Netherlands has fallen from 12.4 per 100 000 in 1960–4 to 7.0 in 1980–4. The fact that mortality has been decreasing since 1960, suggests that other factors are at least partly responsible for this, although screening may have led to an increased rate of fall after 1975.

A number of authors have attempted to demonstrate the effectiveness of cervical screening by case-control studies [3, 14, 17, 45, 60, 66, 78]. However, such analyses are hampered by selection bias [53], and this is likely to be particularly true in the case of cervical screening, where women at the highest risk of disease may be those least likely to respond to invitations for screening. In some of these studies, attempts have been made to take account of selection bias by adjusting for known risk factors also likely to be associated with compliance. However, such adjustments rarely alter the estimated relative risk to the extent which would be expected. These studies are also subject to other biases due to selection of controls, and problems with differentiating between screening and symptomatic smears. Thus, although these studies lend support to the hypothesis that screening is effective, they provide little useful evidence of the degree of benefit. The relative risks from such studies in women ever screened compared with the never screened range from 0.10 to 0.37. The published studies are summarised in Table 2.1 (opposite) (from [53]).

The Effectiveness of Screening in the UK

In the United Kingdom, screening for cervical cancer has been widely available since the mid-1960s, but poorly organised, with a large proportion of smears being taken in the young age-groups, and with low-risk women being screened repeatedly, whereas those at high risk remained unscreened. By 1985, around 3 million smears were being taken a year, with no obvious resulting fall in mortality [44]. However, until recently the programme has lacked any cohesive organisation, with smears being taken, often "opportunistically" at a variety of locations, including family planning clinics, antenatal clinics and GP surgeries. The result has been that a large proportion of smears were taken in the youngest age-group least at risk, and that while some women were screened repeatedly at short intervals, a number remained unscreened. Problems with inadequate follow-up of women with abnormal smears have also contributed to the system's lack of effectiveness. It has been suggested that, with evidence of increasing trends in incidence of cervical cancer in younger women, screening in fact may have prevented an increase which would otherwise have occurred [19]. However, a study comparing registration rates and smear-taking in the 14 English regions, Wales, Scotland and England failed to demonstrate a significant correlation between regional smear rate and age-specific outcome measures, although there was a correlation between screening effect and age-adjusted mortality [54]. It has also been shown that the majority of cases of invasive cancer occur in women who have never previously been screened [25].

Evidence that screening can be effective within the UK is provided by data from parts of Scotland, such as the Grampian region, where an organised screening programme based on the central pathology laboratory in Aberdeen was set up in 1960. A marked decrease in the incidence of invasive cervical cancer compared with the rest of Scotland has been shown, the standardised incidence ratio for Aberdeen city compared with the rest of Scotland falling from over 100% to below 50% [50].

By the mid-1980s, the need for an organised screening programme, on the basis of evidence from the UK and elsewhere was recognised, and a systematic programme of call and recall was introduced, based on the computerised register held by Family Health Service Authorities. Most districts are now offering 3-yearly screening to all women over age 25 years, and there are recent indications that this systematic approach is now starting to achieve a reduction in mortality [69].

The UK is not the only country where a substantial level of screening has failed to achieve the reduction in mortality that might be expected. In Belgium, despite an attempt in the 1960s to screen all women over age 21 years, coverage was poor, and screening has failed to have any impact on trends in mortality or incidence [23]. Likewise in New Zealand, the unorganised nature of the screening programme has been thought to be responsible for its lack of effectiveness, but it has also been

Table 2.1 Case-control studies of cervical screening (from [53])

	Toronto	Netherlands	Maryland	California	Milan	Geneva	Denmark
Screening introduced		1976		Late 1960s		1962–	1968
Cases diagnosed in	1973-6	1979-85 (Aged <70 years)	1982-84	1977-1981 + cases diagnosed 1971-1976 currently under treatment/observation	1981-3	1970-6	1983
Matching of controls	Age, neighbourhood, type of dwelling	Age, district	Age, race, neighbourhood	Age, neighbourhood	Age	Age, nationality, civil status	Age, area
% cases screened	32%	47%		4%	31%	18%	45%
% controls screened	56%	68%		31%	64%	38%	67%
Definition of screening history	"Screening" smears 12-72 months before diagnosis	"Preventive" smears 12+ months before diagnosis	Screened within 3 years	"Screening" smears 12-72 months before diagnosis	"Screening" smears	Negative smears 0-120 months before diagnosis	6+ months before diagnosis
Relative risk of invasive cancer (ever versus never screened)	0.37	0.32	0.29	0.10	0.26	0.31	0.25

suggested that, as in the UK, screening has prevented a greater increase in incidence and mortality than has been observed [20].

The Treatment of Screen-Detected Lesions

Although there is general agreement that cases of moderate or severe dyskaryosis require further investigation, the management of women found to have mild dyskaryosis remains the subject of debate. In 1986, a UK Intercollegiate Working Party concluded that, although the optimum management was uncertain, even women with evidence of mild or moderate dyskaryosis should be referred for immediate colposcopy, although it was acknowledged that in practice this would result in an unacceptable increase in workload for colposcopy clinics [68]. A number of authors, however, believe that such a policy is too aggressive [24, 30, 39]. This opinion is based on evidence that a large proportion of cases of mild dyskaryosis would not progress to severe dyskaryosis or invasive cancer if left untreated. However, a study in Aberdeen, in which women presenting with a mildly or moderately dyskaryotic smear were randomised to different periods of cytological follow-up before biopsy, concluded that cytological surveillance, although safe, was inefficient because of the small proportion of women who benefited by not eventually requiring treatment [28].

In the absence of any data from controlled trials, follow-up studies in areas with different management policies provide the best information on the likely outcomes. Ellman [24] summarised three studies in which patients with mild or moderate dyskaryosis were followed by repeat smears only. These data suggest that around 60% of such lesions will regress to normal, with approximately 15% progressing to severe dyskaryosis within 2–4 years. Jones et al. [38] carried out a study in two districts, one of which had a policy of early colposcopy and the other one of cytological surveillance; in both districts women with mild dyskaryosis were followed-up for an average of 27–32 months and then referred for colposcopy. In the group followed by cytological surveillance, 38% were found to be disease-free on colposcopy, and 12% were found to have CIN3, compared with the early colposcopy group in which 63% were disease-free and none had CIN3.

The costs which need to be borne in mind when considering the optimum policy are not just the risk of "missed" cases compared with the financial cost of increased colposcopy. Referral for colposcopy may lead to greater anxiety among these women than among those that are recalled for repeat smears, as well as resulting in increased treatment in a number of cases. However, the "failures" of non-referral will always be given a high level of publicity, and this creates a climate in which conservative follow-up is difficult to promote. Perhaps the best way forward is for women to be increasingly informed of the potential hazards and benefits, and encouraged to become involved in the decision-making process, in a similar way to that now being used in decisions on the management of breast cancer.

There are now a number of alternative forms of colposcopic treatment available for CIN. These cases considered suitable for conservative treatment are in general those in which the transformation zone can be completely visualised. Most methods of conservative treatment involve physical destruction of the lesion. They include cryotherapy, in which the area is frozen using probes to apply carbon dioxide or nitrous oxide; electrodiathermy, and "cold" coagulation in which heat is used to destroy the tissue; and laser therapy. More recently, the use of loop diathermy excision has become more widespread. This has the advantage that it is relatively cheap, and can be performed on an outpatient basis; also, since it is an excisional as opposed to an ablative technique, it will provide material for histology and thus allow patients to be diagnosed and treated at first outpatient attendance [47].

All the above forms of treatment are associated with post-treatment side-effects to a varying degree, and also with the possibility of persistent CIN following treatment.

In cases of CIN where the entire lesion cannot be visualised, cone biopsy or, more rarely, hysterectomy is carried out.

Cost-Effectiveness of Cervical Screening

Estimates of the cost of saving a life through cervical screening vary widely, even within the UK [16]. Most economic evaluations of cervical screening have been cost-effectiveness analyses, measuring life-years gained and financial cost only. Of more interest, perhaps, is the effect of marginal changes in screening policy, such as changes in the screening frequency, or variation in the minimum and maximum ages at which screening should be offered [12].

Frequency of Cervical Screening

Screening programmes in different countries to date have employed varying recommended screening intervals, and within any programme the actual interval between screens will vary from that recommended. A collaborative study carried out by the International Agency for Research on Cancer has used the data available from different screening programmes to estimate the risk of invasive disease associated with different screening histories, by looking at the incidence of invasive cancer following a negative cervical smear. This information can then be used to form recommendations for screening policies [36].

The study found less variation between centres in the results following two or more smears than following a single smear, suggesting that the sensitivity of screening may vary between programmes but that the underlying disease natural history is a common factor. The results following two or more smears showed a relative protection of 15.3 at 0–11 months following a negative smear, falling to 1.6 at 7–9 years. These results translate to an estimated 91.4% reduction in the cumulative rate of invasive disease up to age 64 years, with three-yearly screening, with little additional benefit associated with more frequent screening. However, these are the reductions that would be achieved with 100% compliance. The IARC study found five-yearly screening giving a protection of 83.7% to be most cost-effective. Nevertheless, three-yearly screening is usually recommended where resources permit [81] but more frequent screening than this is very difficult to justify.

Minimum Age for Screening

Increases in the incidence of cervical cancer among young women have led to a reduction in the lower age at which screening is offered in a number of countries. There have been suggestions that the disease is more rapidly progressive in younger women, and therefore that screening, say below age 30 years, should be conducted more frequently. However, evidence for this more rapid progression is largely anecdotal, and the observations can be explained by other factors [72]. Since the increased incidence observed in young women is almost certainly a cohort effect, which will increase further as they get older, it is essential that in future younger women are not screened at the expense of those older women more at risk.

Maximum Age for Screening

There is some dispute over the upper age limit at which screening should be offered. It has been suggested recently that for women aged over 50 years with a history of negative smears, screening may safely be discontinued [79]. However, screening will still be of value in women aged over 60 years who have never been screened, although the potentially low uptake of screening in older women has led some to question its cost-effectiveness. It has been suggested that screening of women over 65 years could result in a significant reduction in mortality merely by resulting in diagnosis of invasive cancer at an earlier stage [29].

The costs involved in cervical screening are, however, not all financial. The anxiety caused in women with an abnormal smear result has not been widely studied. It has been shown that some diagnosed with CIN [13] are adversely affected psycho-sexually. However, a woman may also be recalled for other reasons such as an insufficient sample, laboratory error (such as a lost or broken slide) or non-significant infection as well as for abnormalities requiring further investigation and/or treatment. While anxiety in such women is likely to be fairly transient, it would seem appropriate to attempt to minimize the period of anxiety.

Quality Control Issues

The essential factors in ensuring the success of a cervical screening programme appear to be central organisation and quality control. The latter should extend to all elements of the screening process – including identification of the population at risk, taking the smear, reading the smear and the follow-up of abnormal smears. Failures of various parts of this process have received widespread publicity in recent years.

Smear Taking

It is not necessary for the person taking the smear to be medically qualified, and in some countries paramedical staff take many of the smears. It is widely accepted that for a smear to be adequate, endocervical cells must be present, as an indicator that the correct region has been sampled. Inadequate smears, or those that cannot be satisfactorily read because of coexisting infection, should be repeated as soon as possible (in the latter case after the infection has been treated).

Reading of Smears

Cervical smears can be read by cytotechnicans, who are trained to look for abnormalities associated with CIN or dysplasia. There are variations in protocol as to whether or not coincidental infection is reported. Quality control of the smear reading process usually involves some form of double reading of a sample of slides.

Follow-up of Abnormals

It has been found that among a sample of cases of invasive cancer, 68% had never been screened and that 13% had had an abnormal smear which had been inadequately followed-up [25]. The need for some "fail-safe" mechanism to avoid such occurrences is now widely recognised [15], although not always successfully implemented.

Sensitivity of Screening

The sensitivity of cervical screening has been studied both by comparison of the relative sensitivity of different techniques or repeat cytology carried out simultaneously, or by identification of cases of invasive cervical cancer in women previously screened negative. Comparison of the different estimates is hampered by variation in the criteria used [52]. A study by Frisch et al. [31], in which patients with only inflammatory smears were colposcoped, estimated the sensitivity of a cytological diagnosis of CIN as only 20%, which increased to 51% with duplicate reading at another laboratory. Similar estimates have been obtained elsewhere, and this low sensitivity has led to some calls for a second smear to be taken at a shorter than routine interval after the first. A study by Giles et al. [32] in which 200 asymptomatic women were screened by cytology and colposcopy found no false negative cytology for cases with histologic CIN3, but 60% and 31% false negative rates for histologic CIN2 and CIN1, respectively. In the Netherlands a population-based study estimated the sensitivity of screening for carcinoma in situ or invasive carcinoma to be 83% [78].

False negative cytology may result from failure of one of a number of parts of the system outlined above [52].

Potential for Automation

There is a clear potential for an automated process of interpretation of cervical smears, if this could be achieved without loss of accuracy. Research is taking place into methods of mechanically obtaining optical data from slides and the computer analysis of such data. Another approach is that of flow cytometry, which can potentially be used for discrimination between neoplastic and non-neoplastic cells.

Alternative Tests

The use of self-collected specimens has been suggested by a number of researchers as being particularly suitable for screening in remote districts with few medical personnel. The major problems with such techniques appear to be failure to collect adequate cells, and the degeneration of specimens prior to analysis. A method has been suggested, which aims to overcome these difficulties by use of a sponge which is inserted into the vagina and rotated to absorb cells, and is then immediately fixed in ethyl alcohol, and can be mailed to a laboratory. Preliminary results suggest the method may detect as many abnormalities as cytology smears, although disagreeing in the degree of severity [57]. However, no data are available from any large-scale trial.

Cervicography was first proposed as a screening technique by Stafl in 1981 [75]. It is a non-invasive procedure which involves taking photographs of the cervix, which is first exposed to 5% acetic acid, using a cervicograph camera. The film is developed and the cervicogram then projected, giving an image for evaluation which is comparable to direct visual colposcopy, by which areas of abnormal epithelium can be identified. Stafl claimed that cervicography should give similar results to colposcopy, which is not practical as an initial screening test because of its cost, and the need for expert evaluation.

Tawa et al. [77] compared the performance of the Pap smear and cervicography in a series of 3271 patients each of whom had both screening tests, the results of which were assessed independently. Among patients found positive by either test, the cervicogram was significantly more sensitive than the Pap smear (14/81 vs 72/81) ($p < 0.001$). However, the smear was significantly more specific than the cervicogram (3165/3190 vs 2889/3190). There was also a much higher percentage of unsatisfactory cervicograms than of Pap smears. However, the authors calculated that cervicography would be more cost-effective as a screening tool, detecting 3.7 times more CIN per dollar than the Pap smear.

Screening in Developing Countries

Despite the impact of screening on cervical cancer in much of the developed world, the disease remains the third most common cancer in the world, with three-quarters of all cases occurring in developing countries, where cervical cancer is the commonest cancer in women.

About 16% of total cases in the world each year occur in India, where age-standardised incidence rates of between 15 and 46 per 100000 have been reported. For the Southern Asian region the crude incidence rate was estimated to be 21.2 per 100000 in 1985 [63]. The disease is noticeably more common in Hindu women than in Muslims. The arguments concerning cost-effectiveness of screening are clearly of more crucial importance in developing countries, where resources are scarce. Attempts to introduce screening have been made in some developing countries. In India, some screening has been taking place since the early 1960s, both through institutions such as outpatient clinics and antenatal clinics and at a community level, using mobile cancer detection units and cancer detection camps. For example, population screening in a rural area has been organised from the Regional Cancer Centre at Trivandrum since 1978, and has reported prevalence rates of malignancy of 3.1 per 1000 women screened [48].

However, in most developing countries only a small proportion of women are reached by screening programmes. To some extent the earlier problems experienced in the UK are being repeated, with young women, identified through family planning clinics, being repeatedly screened at the expense of older women more at risk.

The difficulties facing attempts to introduce screening in developing countries include the fact that the problems of communicable diseases have largely overshadowed that of cancer, leading to little allocation of finances for cancer control. It is not only financial resources that are limited in developing countries, but the human resources needed to run a screening programme, with a lack of trained cytopathologists, cytotechnologists and cytotechnicians, and also the availability of facilities for follow-up and treatment of referrals. Even if the resource problems were overcome, social attitudes would need to alter to establish compliance with any screening programme.

Against this background, it has been suggested for some time that the minimum age for screening should be increased to 35 years, in order to cover women most at risk, and that the screening interval should be increased to as much as 10 years in order to maximise the population covered [76].

A WHO meeting report [81] which summarised the priorities for screening in developing countries, identified the primary aim as being to screen every woman once in her lifetime between the ages of 35 and 40, with screening every 10 years been 35 and 55 where resources are available. Although more frequent screening or commencing screening at younger ages would be preferable, it was stressed that screening should only be carried out within the capabilities of both diagnostic and therapeutic resources available. It has recently been estimated, using data from three Indian cancer registries, that once-only screening offered at age 45 years could reduce the cumulative incidence rate of invasive cervical cancer by 20%–27%, and would be more cost-effective than a single screen at earlier ages [55].

An alternative strategy that has been proposed for developing countries is the use of direct visual inspection of the cervix. It has been suggested that, although this would not decrease the incidence of invasive disease by detecting precancerous lesions, it might result in detection of invasive disease at an earlier stage, and thus decrease mortality. A study of 44970 women attending maternal and child health centres in Delhi with minor symptoms detected 238 cancers, a prevalence of 5.3 per

1000 [73]. However, it has been argued that because these women were symptomatic this does not reflect a true screening situation, and that further training, resources and education would be required to implement a screening programme using this method [33, 74].

The Role of HPV in Cervical Cancer

Evidence has been accumulating for a considerable time that a sexually transmitted agent is associated, probably causally, with invasive cervical cancer. In the 1970s, it was widely believed that the herpes simplex virus was the likely agent, but more recent studies have failed to provide support for this hypothesis.

Human papillomavirus (HPV) now appears to be the most likely aetiological factor and types 16 and 18 in particular have been found to be linked to invasive cervical cancer. Development of molecular biology techniques, in particular polymerase chain reaction (PCR), have made it feasible to identify type-specific DNA on a large scale.

However, the high prevalence of HPV found in normal samples, particularly in young women, has until recently cast some doubt on the hypothesis. A study of samples from normal women in Greenland and Denmark found a higher prevalence of HPV 16 and 18 in Denmark than in Greenland, despite the fact that the latter has a 5–6-fold higher incidence rate of cervical cancer [41].

Improvements in the quality of PCR, however, have led to more accurate studies, and it has been recently shown that a number of HPV types, including not only 16 and 18 but others such as 33 and 35 are linked to CIN2–3 and invasive cervical cancer, with a wider range of subtypes associated with CIN1. It has been suggested that there is thus a potential use of HPV testing in deciding which cases of CIN1 are likely to progress and require immediate treatment as opposed to those which can be allocated a more conservative follow-up [7]. These findings may also have implications for the development of vaccines both for the treatment and, eventually, the prevention of cervical cancer.

References

1. Aareleid T, Pukkali E, Thomson H, Hakama M (1993) Cervical cancer incidence and mortality trends in Finland and Estonia: a screened vs an unscreened population. Eur J Cancer 29A:745–749.
2. Ahluwalia MS, Doll R (1968) Mortality from cancer of the cervix in British Columbia and other parts of Canada. Br J Prev Soc Med 22:161–164.
3. Aristazabel N, Cuello C, Correa P, Collazos T, Haenzel W (1984) The impact of vaginal cytology on cervical cancer risk in Cali, Colombia. Int J Cancer 34:5–9.
4. Ayre JE (1947) Selective cytology smear for diagnosis of cancer. Am J Obstet Gynecol 53:609–617.

5. Babes A (1928) Diagnostic du cancer du col uterin par les frattis. Presse Med 36:451–454.

6. Barton SE, Jenkins D, Cuzick J, Maddox PH, Edwards R, Singer A (1988) Effect of cigarette smoking on cervical epithelial immunity. Lancet ii:652–654.

7. Beral V, Day NE (1992) Screening for cervical cancer: is there a place for incorporating tests for the human papillomavirus? In: Munoz N, Bosch FX, Shah KV, Meheus A (eds) The epidemiology of cervical cancer and human papillomavirus. IARC, Lyon, pp 263–269.

8. Boyes DA, Morrison B, Knox EG et al. (1982) A cohort study of cervical cancer screening in British Columbia. Clin Investigative Med 5:1–29.

9. Brinton LA, Fraumeni F Jr (1986) Epidemiology of uterine cervical cancer. J Chron Dis 39:1051.

10. Brinton LA, Reeves WC, Brenes MM et al. (1989) The male factor in the etiology of cervical cancer among sexually monogamous women. Int J Cancer 44:199–203.

11. Brinton LA, Reeves WC, Brenes MM et al. (1990) Oral contraceptive use and risk of invasive cervical cancer. Int J Cancer 19:4–11.

12. Brown J, Sculpher MJ (1993) Economics of screening programmes to prevent cervical cancer. Contemp Rev Gynaecol 5:221–229.

13. Campion MJ, Brown JR, McCance DJ et al. (1988) Psychosexual trauma of an abnormal cervical smear. Br J Obstet Gynaecol 95:175–181.

14. Celantano D, Klassen A, Weiseman C, Rosenhein N (1988) Cervical cancer screening practices among older women: results from the Maryland cervical cancer case-control study. J Clin Epidemiol 41:531–541.

15. Chamberlain J, Pike C (1991) Fail-safe actions to ensure follow-up investigation of women with abnormal cytology; Guidelines. NHS Cervical Screening Programme. Muir Gray, Oxford.

16. Charny MC, Farrow SC, Roberts CJ (1987) The cost of saving a life through cervical cytology screening: implications for health policy. Health Policy 7:345–359.

17. Clarke EA, Anderson TW (1979) Does screening by "Pap" smears help prevent cervical cancer? A case-control study. Lancet ii:1–4.

18. Coppleson LW, Brown B (1975) Observation on a model of the biology of carcinoma of the cervix. A poor fit between observation and theory. Am J Obstet Gynecol 122:127–136.

19. Cook GA, Draper GJ (1984) Trends in cervical cancer and carcinoma in-situ in Great Britain. Br J Cancer 50:367–375.

20. Cox B, Skegg DCG (1992) Projections of cervical cancer mortality and incidence in New Zealand: the possible impact of screening. J Epidemiol Community Health 46:373–377.

21. Cramer D (1974) The role of cervical cytology in the declining morbidity and mortality from cervical cancer. Cancer 34:2018–2027.

22. Cuzick J, Boyle P (1988) Trends in cervix cancer mortality. Cancer Surveys 7:417–439.

23. De Schryver A (1989) Does screening for cervical cancer affect incidence and mortality trends? The Belgian Experience. Eur J Clin Oncol 25:395–399.

24. Ellman R (1991) Indications for colposcopy from a UK viewpoint. In: Miller AB, Day NE, Chamberlain J, Day NE, Hakama M, Prorok PC (eds) Cancer screening. UICC project of evaluation of screening for cancer. Cambridge University Press, Cambridge, pp 257–183.

25. Ellman R, Chamberlain J (1984) Improving the effectiveness of cervical cancer screening. J R Coll Gen Pract 34:537–542.

26. Evaluation Committee (1989) Population screening for cervical cancer in the Netherlands. Int J Epidemiol 18:775-781.

27. Evans DMD, Hudson EA, Brown CL et al. (1986) Terminology in gynaecological cytopathology: report of the Working Party of the British Society for Clinical Cytology. J Clin Pathol 39:933-944.

28. Flannelly G, Anderson D, Kitchener HC et al. (1994) Management of women with mild and moderate cervical dyskaryosis. Br Med J 308:1399-1403.

29. Fletcher A (1990) Screening for cancer of the cervix in elderly women. Lancet 335:97-99.

30. Fletcher A, Metaxas N, Grubb C, Chamberlain J (1990) Four and a half year follow-up of women with dyskaryotic cervical smears. Br Med J 301:641-644.

31. Frisch LE, Parmar H, Buckley LD, Chalem SA (1990) Improving the sensitivity of cervical cytologic screening. A comparison of duplicate smears and colposcopic examination of patients with cytologic inflammatory epithelial changes. Acta Cytologica 34:136-139.

32. Giles JA, Hudson E, Crow J, Williams D, Walker P (1988) Colposcopic assessment of the accuracy of cervical cytology screening. Br Med J 296:1099-1102.

33. Griffiths M (1992) Screening for cervical cancer in developing countries. Br Med J 304:984.

34. Greenberg RS, Chow W, Liff JM (1989) Recent trends in the epidemiology of cervical neoplasia. Acta Cytol 33:463-469.

35. Habbema JDF, Lubbe JTN, van Oortmarssen GJ, van der Maas PJ (1987) A simulation approach to cost-effectiveness and cost-benefit calculations for early detection of disease. Eur J Op Res 29:159-166.

36. IARC Working Group on Evaluation of Cervical Cancer Screening Programmes (1986) Screening for squamous cervical cancer: duration of low risk after negative results of cervical cytology and its implication for screening policies. Br Med J 293:659-664.

37. Johannesson G, Geirsson G, Day N (1978) The effect of mass screening in Iceland, 1965-1974, on the incidence of cervical carcinoma. Int J Cancer 21:418-425.

38. Jones MH, Jenkins D, Cuzick J et al. (1992) Mild cervical dyskariosis: safety of cytological surveillance. Lancet 339:1440-1443.

39. Kirby AJ, Spiegelhalter DJ, Day NE et al. (1992) Conservative treatment of mild/moderate cervical dyskariosis: long-term outcome. Lancet 339:828-831.

40. Kjellgren O (1986) Mass screening in Sweden for cancer of the uterine cervix: effect on incidence and mortality. An overview. Gyncecol abstract. Lancet 22:56-63.

41. Kjaer SK, de Villiers E-M, Haugaard BJ et al. (1988) Human papillomavirus, herpes simplex virus and cervical cancer incidence in Greenland and Denmark. A population-based cross-sectional study. Int J Cancer 41:518-524.

42. Knox EG (1973) A simulation system for screening procedures. In: McLachlan G (ed) The future and present initiatives. (Problems and progress in medical care IX.) Nuffield Provincial Hospitals Trust, Oxford, pp 19-30.

43. Kuroishi T, Hirose K, Tominaga S (1986) Evaluation of the efficacy of mass screening for uterine cancer in Japan. Japan J Cancer Res 77:399-405.

44. Lancet (1985) (editorial) Death by incompetence. Lancet ii:363-364.

45. La Vecchia C, Franceschi S, Decarli A et al. (1984) "Pap" smear and the risk of cervical neoplasia; quantitative estimates from a case-control study. Lancet ii:779-782.

46. Louhivouri K (1991) Effect of a mass screening programme on the risk of cervical cancer. Cancer Detect Prev 15:471-474.

47. Luesley DM, Cullimore J, Redman CWE et al. (1990) Loop diathermy excision of the

cervical transformation zone in patients with abnormal cervical smears. Br Med J 300:1690–1693.

48. Luthra UK, Rengachari R (1986) Organization of screening programmes in developing countries with reference to screening for cancer of the uterine cervix in India. In: Hakama M, Miller AB, Day NE (eds) Screening for cancer of the uterine cervix. IARC, Lyon, pp 273–285.

49. Lynge E, Madsen M, Engholm G (1989) Effect of organised screening on incidence and mortality of cervical cancer in Denmark. Cancer Res 49:2157–2160.

50. MacGregor JE, Moss SM, Parkin DM, Day NE (1986) Cervical cancer screening in north-east Scotland. In: Hakama M, Miller AB, Day NE (eds) Screening for cancer of the uterine cervix. IARC, Lyon, pp 25–36.

51. Miller AB, Lindsay J, Hill GB (1976) Mortality from cancer of the uterus in Canada and its relationship to screening for cancer of the cervix. Int J Cancer 17:602–612.

52. Modan B (1993) Screening for cervical cancer – should the routine be challenged? Eur J Cancer 29A:2320–2325.

53. Moss SM (1991) Case-control studies of screening. Int J Epidemiol 20:1–6.

54. Murphy MFG, Campbell MJ, Goldblatt PO (1987) Twenty years' screening of the uterine cervix in Great Britain, 1964–84: further evidence for its ineffectiveness. J Epidemiol Community Health 42:49–53.

55. Murthy NS, Agarwal S, Prabhakar AK, Sharma S, Das DK (1993) Estimation of reduction in life-time risk of cervical cancer through one life-time screening. Neoplasma 40:255–258.

56. Narod SA, Thompson DW, Jain M et al. (1991) Dysplasia and the natural history of cervical cancer: early results of the Toronto cohort study. Eur J Cancer 27:1141–1416.

57. Noguchi M, Nakanishi M, Kato K (1982) Appraisal of a newly developed self-collection device for obtaining cervical specimens. Acta Cytologica 26:633–635.

58. Office of Population Censuses and Surveys (1993) Cancer statistics: cause, 1987. Series MB1, no. 20. HMSO, London.

59. Office of Population Censuses and Surveys (1993) Mortality statistics: cause 1992. Series DH2, no. 19. HMSO, London.

60. Olesen F (1988) A case-control study of cervical cytology before diagnosis of cervical cancer in Denmark. Int J Epidemiol 17:501–508.

61. Papanicolaou GM, Traut HF (1941) The diagnostic value of vaginal smears in carcinoma of the uterus. Am J Obstet and Gynecol 42:193–206.

62. Parkin DM (1985) A computer simulation model for the practical planning of cervical cancer screening programmes. Br J Cancer 51:551–568.

63. Parkin DM, Pisani P, Ferlay J (1993) Estimates of the worldwide incidence of eighteen major cancers in 1985. Int J Cancer 54:594–606.

64. Pedersen E, Haeg K, Kolstad P (1971) Mass screening for cancer of the uterine cervix in Ostfold County, Norway. An experiment. Acta Obstet Gynecol Scand Suppl 11.

65. Pisani P, Parkin DM, Ferlay J (1993) Estimates of the worldwide mortality from eighteen major cancers in 1985. Implications for prevention and projections of future burden. Int J Cancer 55:891–903.

66. Raymond L, Obradovic M, Riotton G (1984) A case-control study to estimate the detection of cancer of the cervix uteri by cytology. Rev Epidemiol Sante Publique 32:10–15.

67. Robertson AJ, Anderson JM, Swanson Beck J et al. (1989) Observer variablility in the histopathological reporting of cervical biopsies. J Clin Pathol 42:231–238.

68. Royal College of Obstetricians and Gynaecologists (1987) Report of the Intercollegiate

Working Party on Cervical Cancer Screening. Royal College of Obstetricians and Gynecologists, London.

69. Sasieni P (1991) Trends in cervical cancer mortality. Lancet 338:818–819.
70. Schiffman MH, Bauer HM, Hoover RN et al. (1993) Epidemiologic evidence showing that human papilloma virus infection causes most cervical intraepithelial neoplasia. J Natl Cancer Instit 85:958–964.
71. Sigurdsson K (1993) Effect of organised screening on the risk of cervical cancer. Evaluation of screening activity in Iceland. Int J Cancer 54:563–570.
72. Silcocks PBS, Moss SM (1988) Rapidly progressive cervical cancer: is it a real problem? Br J Obstet and Gynaecol 95:1111–1116.
73. Singh V, Sehgal A, Luthra UK (1992) Screening for cervical cancer by direct inspection. Br Med J 304:534–535.
74. Soe MM (1992) Screening for cervical cancer in developing countries. Br Med J 304:983–984.
75. Stafl A (1981) Cervicography – a new approach to cervical cancer detection. Gynecol Oncol 12:5292–5301.
76. Stjernsward J, Eddy D, Luthra U, Stanley K (1987) Plotting a new course for cervical cancer screening in developing countries. World Health Forum 8:42–45.
77. Tawa K, Forsythe A, Coye K, Saltz A, Peter HW, Watring WG (1988) A comparison of the Papanicolaou smear and the Cervigram: sensitivity, specificity and cost analysis. Obstet Gynecol 71:229–233.
78. van der Graaf Y, Zielhuis G, Peer P, Vooijs P (1988) The effectiveness of cervical screening: a population-based case-control study. J Clin Epidemiol 41:21–26.
79. van Wijngaarden WJ, Duncan ID (1993) Rationale for stopping cervical screening in women over 50. Br Med J 306:967–971.
80. Vessey MP, Lawless M, McPherson K et al. (1983) Neoplasia of the cervix uteri and contraception: a possible adverse effect of the pill. Lancet ii:930–934.
81. World Health Organization Report (1986) Control of cancer of the cervix uteri. Bull World Health Organ 64:607–618.
82. Ziegler RG, Brinton LA, Hamman RF et al. (1990) Diet and the risk of invasive cervical cancer among white women in the United States. Am J Epidemiol 132:432–445.

3 – Screening for Cancer of the Breast

Sue Moss and Jocelyn Chamberlain

Epidemiology

Breast cancer is the most common cancer among women, with an estimated 308 100 cancers worldwide in 1985, accounting for 19.1% of all cancers [62]. It is the most common cancer in women in all developed countries, apart from Japan. The highest recorded incidence rates are in North America, with an age-standardised rate in 1985 of 84.8 per 100 000. The lowest reported rates are 11.1 per 100 000 in Western Africa and 14.6 per 100 000 in China. In England and Wales, the age-standardised incidence rate in 1987 was 58.0 per 100 000, representing 23 740 new cases [59]. Breast cancer in males is rare, and will not be considered further in this chapter.

The lifetime risk of developing breast cancer is now approximately one in 12 in the UK. The incidence of breast cancer increases with age, the disease being rare below age 25. In areas of high incidence there is usually a slower rate of increase around the age of the menopause, and generally a slower rate of increase from age 50 onwards [65]. The resulting plateau in age-specific incidence has led in the past to a hypothesis that breast cancer is actually two distinct diseases [23], but is generally now believed to be the result of the influence of hormones on risk at different ages.

Breast cancer is also the most common cause of death from cancer in women worldwide, again with the highest rates in developed countries other than Japan, although in the United States and in Scotland it has now been overtaken by lung cancer [18]. Estimated age-standardised mortality rates in 1985 ranged from 28.2 per 100 000 in North America and 27.7 per 100 000 in Northern Europe to 4.7 per 100 000 in Eastern Asia [66]. In England and Wales in 1992 there were 13 634 deaths from breast cancer, with an age-standardised rate of 27.7 per 100 000 [58], and at ages 35–54 years it was the leading overall cause of death. Nevertheless, 88% of breast cancer deaths occur in women over age 50 years, and 40% in women over age 75 years.

Within the UK, the incidence of breast cancer appears to have increased slightly between 1980 and 1987, the last year before the national screening programme was introduced. There is already evidence from both the United States and the UK that screening is leading to a further increase in incidence in some age-groups [31].

However, age-specific mortality rates below age 70 years have shown a recent decline in England and Wales, starting before the national screening programme could have had any measurable effect [8], possibly due to advances in treatment.

Aetiology

Hormones

A number of factors point to a key role of endogenous hormones in the aetiology of breast cancer [10]. An increased risk of the disease has been shown by a number of authors to be associated with early age at menarche, late age at first full-term pregnancy or nulliparity and late age at menopause, with relative risks generally of the order of 1.5–2.0 (for example for first birth over age 30 compared to below age 20). There is also some evidence of a protective effect of breast feeding. These factors suggest an increased risk due to exposure to oestrogens, and oestradiol in particular, perhaps in conjunction with progesterone, but the precise mechanism is still the subject of some debate.

The risk due to exogenous hormones from the use of oral contraceptives and hormone replacement therapy is still not clear. There is some evidence that long-term use of oestrogen replacement therapy may result in a slight increase in risk. Most evidence on the use of oral contraceptives suggests an increased risk of breast cancer incidence below age 45 years associated with long-term use, but some studies fail to confirm this. However, more data are needed on the effect of more recent "low dose" pills, and on the risk of long-term use at older ages [77].

Diet

Diet also appears to play a major role in the aetiology of breast cancer, and may be responsible for many of the reported differences between countries and races, in particular the notably low incidence of the disease in Japan. An increased risk has been observed with obesity, and with high dietary fat intake [11]. De Waard and Trichopoulos [24] have suggested that an increased risk of breast cancer may result from an energy rich diet in childhood and adolescence; such a diet is also associated with early menarche. They hypothesise that both nutritional and reproduction factors may act through endocrine mechanisms.

A number of, although not all, studies have shown a fairly weak association between alcohol intake and increasing risk of breast cancer. However, there is a lack of consistency in evidence of dose–response and in the level of intake at which an increased risk becomes apparent. It is possible that age at consumption may be relevant, with an increased risk associated with consumption at young ages. The majority of the evidence on cigarette smoking points to a lack of any effect on risk of breast cancer.

Family History

There is an increased risk of breast cancer in women with a family history of the disease, with a relative risk of 2.0 or more being observed in women with one or more affected first degree relatives. The risk is strongest in women with relatives affected below the age of 50 years [42]. In recent developments one inherited breast cancer gene, BRCA1, has been isolated on chromosome 17 [49], and another one located on chromosome 13 [84], although other genes are probably also involved. In total it is probable that approximately 5% of all breast cancers have a genetic component, the proportion being greater in cases diagnosed at a young age.

Ionising Radiation

Studies of a number of different groups of subjects have provided evidence that ionising radiation can induce breast cancer. These include studies of the atomic bomb survivors [76], and of women who received large doses of radiation for a variety of medical reasons [22, 41]. The risk appears greatest in women irradiated at young ages. However, the majority of the data are derived from women subjected to high doses, making it difficult to extrapolate in order to estimate the effect of low-dose radiation. It is suggested that some women, notably those carrying the ataxia telangiectasia (AT) gene, are more susceptible to the effects of radiation [72].

Primary Prevention

Evidence of the effect of hormones on the risk of breast cancer and of the beneficial effect of tamoxifen on survival of breast cancer patients has led to interest in the possible use of a hormonal agent for breast cancer prevention. Trials of tamoxifen are now taking place in a number of centres – these are mainly restricted to high risk women due to concerns about possible side effects [16]. Similarly, a dietary intervention study in which high-risk women are randomised to a very low fat diet or to a control group is starting as part of the Women's Health Initiative in the US [38] and a prototype contraceptive agent with a gonadotropin-releasing hormone agonist is being piloted [70].

Treatment, Survival and Prognosis of Breast Cancer

The four types of treatment available for patients with breast cancer are surgery, radiotherapy, hormone therapy and chemotherapy. The majority of cases are treated by surgery, usually with one of the other modalities as adjuvant therapy. Radical mastectomy has largely been replaced by simple mastectomy, and there is increasing use of local excision of small tumours. A recent overview of trials of adjuvant hormone therapy and chemotherapy in early breast cancer found a 17%

mortality reduction owing to the use of tamoxifen, and 16% from the use of chemotherapy [28]. Chemotherapy is now sometimes used prior to surgery, and this neoadjuvant therapy has implications for the staging of tumours, since it will result in tumour shrinkage and hence smaller histological measurements.

Overall 5-year survival for breast cancers diagnosed in the UK in the 1980s approaches 65% [13], but it is well known that both local and metastatic recurrences can present very many years after treatment of the primary. Haybittle [40] reviewed the long-term survival of several series of breast cancer patients and noted that even after 35 years the death rate exceeded that of an age-matched normal population. Nevertheless taking into account changes in stage at diagnosis and improvements in adjuvant therapy, he predicted that 40%–50% of patients diagnosed today would not die from their breast cancer.

The survival of patients with breast cancer is largely dependent on the stage of the disease at diagnosis. For cases diagnosed in England and Wales in the period 1981–5 five-year survival of Stage I cases was 84% compared with 18% for Stage IV [18]. There is some variation in reported survival internationally [12], which may in part be due to differences in stage at presentation between countries, and partly due to differences in the completeness of ascertainment of new cases and deaths.

Studies of the long-term survival of breast cancer patients have suggested an increased mortality compared with the general population remaining after 15–20 years [67].

Tumour size, nodal status and histological grade are the most useful indications of prognosis, although histopathologists' classification of tumour by grade is not always consistent. It has been suggested from recent screening data that tumour growth rate may change with time [75].

Tumour size is the single most useful prognostic indicator; there is a close relationship between tumour size and the probability of nodal involvement, but the classification of the latter is dependent on the extent of axillary node sampling undertaken by surgeons. Tumour size probably also correlates closely with the likelihood that the tumour has metastasised [46].

Predisposing Factors

Benign Breast Conditions

A number of benign breast conditions have been implicated as markers for risk of subsequent development of invasive breast cancer. Dupont and Page [26] found women with proliferative benign lesions to have a relative risk of 1.9 compared with those with non-proliferative lesions, whereas those with atypical hyperplasia had a relative risk of 5.3 compared with the same group. The diagnosis of fibroadenoma has been shown recently to be a long-term risk factor for breast cancer, with the risk increased in women with proliferative disease or a family history of breast cancer [27].

The pathological distinction between atypia and carcinoma in situ is subject to considerable observer variation [7]. Two types of carcinoma in situ are recognised, lobular and ductal, of which lobular is the more benign. Ductal carcinoma in situ is generally considered to be a precursor of invasive cancer, being often associated with recurrence at the original site of diagnosis [60]. However, the rate and extent of progression from carcinoma in situ to invasive cancer is still debated.

Mammographic Parenchymal Patterns

In 1976 Wolfe [83] described four distinct mammographic parenchymal patterns, N1, P1, P2 and DY, relating to variations in the mammographic density of breast tissue. N1 patterns indicate that the breast parenchyma is composed of fat, P1 and P2 imply increasing ductal prominence, and DY the presence of nodular densities or dysplasia. Women with DY patterns, and to a lesser extent those with P2, have been shown to be at increased risk of breast cancer compared with those with N or P1. There is considerable variability in the classification of these patterns by radiologists, and it has been suggested that the apparent association is an artefact due to greater difficulty in detecting cancers in dense breasts; however, it is also hypothesised that the effect on risk is due to association of high-risk patterns with high-risk histological changes [37].

The Rationale for Screening

Although the growth rate of breast cancer appears to be very variable, the large difference in stage-specific survival suggests that early detection could be of value in controlling the heavy toll of deaths from this common disease. Moreover, the recent advances in treatment by using adjuvant chemotherapy and tamoxifen are limited to early stage disease; these therapies in Stages III and IV may give temporary remission for several months but are not curative. Therefore, screening and adjuvant treatment are likely to work together, with screening increasing the proportion of patients who are able to benefit from modern treatment methods.

Screening Tests for Breast Cancer

Three principal tests are advocated for detection of presymptomatic breast cancer. They are X-ray mammography, clinical examination (physical examination of the breasts by a trained professional) and breast self-examination (physical examination of the breasts by a woman herself). Some other imaging tests have been tried and found unsatisfactory, such as thermography which lacks both sensitivity and specificity [47], and ultrasound which, although useful in visualising lesions already identified by other tests, lacks sensitivity for very small lesions and is cumbersome to perform in searching the whole breast for possible abnormality [39].

Mammography

Mammography is widely regarded as the optimal test since it is capable not only of detecting lesions as small as 5 mm in diameter, but also can visualise impalpable tumours indicated by the presence of microcalcification or architectural distortion. Typically, of cancers detected by mammography, 17% are lesions in situ and a further 25% are invasive cancers measuring 10 mm or less in diameter [19].

Sensitivity

Several studies have reported on interval cancers following mammographic screening from which estimates of its sensitivity are available. In the Swedish Two-Counties study [75], where screening consisted of just one mediolateral oblique view of each breast, 927 cancers were found by screening, and 76 interval cancers presented within 12 months of a negative screen, giving an estimate of sensitivity of 92%. In Nijmegen in the Netherlands [64], using the same screening method, 305 breast cancers were detected by mammography screening and 67 interval cancers arose in the ensuing 12 months giving a sensitivity of 78%. Some studies such as the Breast Cancer Detection Demonstration Project in the US [6] and the UK Trial of Early Detection of Breast Cancer [55] screened by clinical examination as well as mammography but recorded the findings independently. Taking the sum of interval cancers diagnosed in the 12 months after a negative screen plus those detected by the clinical screen alone as "false negatives" to mammography, the sensitivity of mammography in the US study was 76% and in the UK study 82%.

It is likely that the lead-time gained by mammographic screening is prolonged in some cases and there may be an element of overdiagnosis, particularly among the in situ carcinomas. Therefore inclusion of all mammographically detected tumours in the numerator may give a falsely optimistic estimate of sensitivity. This problem can be overcome by using the proportional incidence method of calculating sensitivity, which, rather than enumerating all cancers detected by screening, calculates the expected number of cancers in successive time periods after a screen whose diagnosis was advanced by screening (see Chapter 1). This not only gives a more realistic estimate of the performance of the screening test, but also shows how sensitivity falls off with time and thus provides evidence on the frequency with which routine screening needs to be repeated. Tabar et al. [73] reported that, in women aged 50–69 years, a single oblique view mammogram of each breast advanced the diagnosis of 87% of breast cancers expected to arise within 12 months of screening, 31% of those expected to arise 12 to 24 months after screening, and 55% of those expected to arise 24–36 months after screening. Similarly, in the UK Trial, Moss et al. [55] found that in 45–64-year-old women the diagnosis had been advanced for 77% of cancers expected within one year of screening by combined mammographic and clinical examination.

Specificity

The proportion of women without breast cancer who required further diagnostic tests because of a suspicious mammogram was 4.4% (specificity 95.6%) in the first round of the Swedish Two-County study, falling to 2% (specificity 98%) in subsequent rounds [75]. Comparable figures from the UK study using clinical examination as well as mammography [79] were specificities of 94% in the first round and 96% in subsequent rounds. The majority of suspicious lesions can be confidently confirmed as non-malignant by relatively non-invasive investigations, including further mammographic views, physical examination, ultrasound, and fine-needle aspiration cytology, so that few women require a biopsy to show that they do not have breast cancer.

No study has assessed the extent to which further mammographic views as part of diagnostic work-up are able to clear suspicious lesions as unimportant, but inclusion of a cephalocaudal as well as mediolateral oblique view in the primary screen has been shown to improve specificity [Wald, personal communication] as well as increasing the cancer detection rate. This is one of the few examples of a measure designed primarily to improve sensitivity which increases, rather than decreases specificity.

Only six per 1000 women without breast cancer required a biopsy for investigation of a suspicious mammogram at the first screen in the Swedish study, falling to less than one per 1000 in subsequent rounds. The increasing use of fine-needle aspiration cytology, under stereotactic control for impalpable lesions, has contributed to reduce biopsy rates [14], and this can be achieved, not merely in research studies but also in widespread application of screening. In the British national screening programme in 1992/93, in the first round 2205 out of 877 000 women without cancer required a biopsy (2 per 1000), falling in the second round to 136 out of 200 000 screened women without cancer (0.6 per 1000). This rate is less than half the rate of benign biopsy in the unscreened control group of the British trial ten years earlier. In North America false positive referral rates and particularly biopsy rates, tend to be higher [31].

Clinical Examination

Although clinical examination may be widely perceived as a suitable test for breast cancer, there have been few studies of its validity. Most screening studies have used it as an adjunct to mammography.

One exception to this is the Canadian National Breast Screening Study in which 19 965 women aged 50–59 years were eligible to receive four or five annual clinical examinations by specially trained nurses or doctors [5]. This was one arm of a randomised trial comparing breast cancer mortality in women screened by clinical examination alone, with that in women screened by clinical examination and mammography. Another relevant study is the UK Trial of Early Detection of Breast Cancer [78] in which women in the screening arm were invited for mammography and clinical examination in rounds 1, 3, 5 and 7, but for clinical examination alone in rounds 2, 4 and 6. The information available from the "clinical only" rounds, however, must be regarded with a certain amount of caution because screening by both modalities 12 months earlier presumably removed some cancers from the pool of those potentially detectable. As in the Canadian study, all the nurses and doctors undertaking clinical examination had undergone special training.

Sensitivity

Taking as the denominator the sum of screen-detected plus interval cancers within 12 months, sensitivity of clinical examination was calculated separately for each year of the Canadian trial and ranged from 57.1% to 83.3%. In the UK trial 74 cancers were detected by the clinical-only screens, and 41 subsequently presented as interval cancers, giving a sensitivity of 66% [55]. This study was also able to calculate sensitivity by the proportional incidence method, using breast cancer incidence in the unscreened control group to derive the expected incidence in the absence of screening. For women aged 45–64 years, 66% of expected cancers were detected by a previous clinical screen, although this is a maximum figure because the possibility that some had already been detected by a combined mammographic plus clinical screen one year earlier cannot be ruled out.

In screening programmes which use a combination of clinical examination and mammography but record their findings independently it is possible to calculate the relative sensitivity of each test, taking all screen-detected cancers as the denominator. One of the earliest screening studies, the HIP trial in New York [69] conducted during the 1960s, reported that out of 132 screen-detected cancers, only 29 (22%) were found by both tests; 59 (45%) were detected by clinical examination but were negative on mammography, whereas 44 (33%) were detected by mammography, but were negative on clinical examination. Developments in mammography since then have resulted in its much greater relative sensitivity and consequent decline in the relative sensitivity of clinical examination. In the US Breast Cancer Detection Demonstration Project during the 1970s, out of 3557 screen-detected cancers, 47.3% were positive to both tests, 41.6% positive on mammography only, and 8.7% positive on clinical examination only (in 2% the detection modality was unknown) [6]. In the UK trial, in the first screening round 67% of 159 cancers were positive to both tests, 29% to mammography alone and 4% to clinical examination alone; comparable proportions for 295 cancers detected in subsequent combined test screening rounds were 45% positive to both, 48% positive to mammography alone and 7% positive to clinical alone. It is findings such as these that have led many health policy makers to conclude that the small extra yield gained by clinical examination does not justify its additional cost. Critics of mammography, however [3, 52, 85], propose that cancers detected by mammography alone are slow-growing biologically non-aggressive neoplasia that do not pose a threat to life, and that, therefore, clinical examination is an equally valid test. However, the fact that the sensitivity of clinical examination using the proportional incidence method (which avoids the possible bias of crediting screening with detection of non-progressive disease) is some 10% lower than that of mammography supports the view that mammography is the superior test.

Specificity of Clinical Examination

The proportion of women without cancer who were referred for diagnostic work-up because of a possible abnormality on physical examination in the Canadian trial ranged from 10.8% at the first screen (specificity 89.2%) to 3.5% at the fifth screen (specificity 96.5%) [51]. The proportion undergoing biopsy which revealed only benign disease was less than 1%, and again fell with each successive screen from 0.9% at the first screen to 0.3% at the fifth screen. In the UK trial [79], during the clinical examination-only rounds, 5% of women without cancer were referred for diagnostic work-up (specificity 95%), and the proportion biopsied was 0.1%–0.25%. Thus it seems that there is little difference between mammography and clinical examination in specificity when estimated from false positive referrals; but clinical examination results in fewer benign biopsies than mammography. Nevertheless, because the cancer detection rate of mammography is greater the predictive value of a positive mammogram is generally higher than that of a positive clinical examination.

Effectiveness of Screening in Reducing Mortality

The effectiveness of screening has been more thoroughly researched for breast cancer than for any other cancer site. No fewer than eight randomised controlled trials, with breast cancer mortality as their end-point, have been conducted [1, 2, 34, 50, 51, 57, 69, 74]. Their findings are augmented by one prospective geographical comparison between populations offered or not offered screening [80], three case-control studies [21, 61, 81] and one demonstration project [53].

The first trial, started in New York in the 1960s, was conducted in a population registered for all medical care in a Health Insurance Plan; membership of the plan was provided for families of employees by several large organisations as a benefit negotiated by trade unions, and the membership represented a balanced cross-section of the New York population. Women aged 40–64 years were randomised into an intervention group, who were offered screening by mammography and clinical examination on four occasions at annual intervals, or into a control group. After 10 years there were 29% fewer breast cancer deaths in the intervention group than the control group, falling to a 21% reduction at an 18-year follow-up. Several trials have been conducted in Sweden. The first, known as the Two-County study, enrolled 133 000 women aged 40–74 years living in the counties of Kopparberg and Ostergotland, and randomised them by parish into an intervention group and a control group. Women in the intervention parishes were offered screening by single-view mammography at an average interval of 33 months for those over 50 years and 24 months for those aged 40–49 years. After 11 years there were 22% fewer breast cancer deaths in the intervention group [75]. Three further randomised controlled trials were conducted in Sweden; in Malmo after 9 years there were 19% fewer deaths in the intervention group, in Stockholm, after 7 years 24% fewer deaths and in Gothenburg, after 5 years 19% fewer deaths [57]. In Edinburgh, general practices were randomised to intervention or control groups; women aged

45 to 64 in the intervention group were invited for clinical breast examination every year, with mammography in alternate years. After 10 years there were 15% fewer deaths in the intervention group [1].

All these trials compared women who were offered screening with a control group not offered screening. Their findings are summarised in Table 3.1 which also shows the 95% confidence intervals around the point estimates of mortality reduction. From this it can be seen that, although all point in the same direction, i.e. lower mortality, only the first two are statistically significant, but some of the later trials lack power due to their relatively small populations and/or short periods of follow-up. When cumulative breast cancer mortality since entry to the trial is plotted separately for intervention and control groups, there is always a time-lag of at least 4 years before mortality in the intervention group starts to diverge from the control group.

Table 3.1   Summary of randomised trials with an unscreened control group

Trial [reference]	Size of intervention group	Years since entry to trial	Relative risk of breast cancer death	95% CI
New York [69]	31 000	18	0.79	0.62–0.99
Two-County [75]	77 000	11	0.78	0.65–0.93
Malmo [2]	21 000	9	0.81	0.62–1.07
Stockholm [34]	39 000	7	0.76	0.50–1.14
Gothenburg [57]	21 000	5	0.81	0.50–1.29
Edinburgh [1]	23 000	10	0.85	0.65–1.12

Two statistical overviews of these trials have been published. The first [57] re-analysed data from the Swedish trials, using a standard end-point and with an independent committee reviewing all relevant deaths. The conclusion of this overview was that the relative risk of breast cancer death in intervention populations compared to controls was 0.77 (95% CI 0.67–0.88). Wald et al. [82] included the New York and Edinburgh findings as well as the Swedish trials in a meta-analysis using only published data from each trial, and found a relative risk of 0.78 (95% CI 0.70–0.87).

The Canadian trials were not included in these meta-analyses because their objectives and design were rather different; both randomised volunteer populations and their control groups were partially screened. The trial in women aged 40–49 years is discussed further below. That in women aged 50–59 years aimed to show whether annual mammography and clinical examination resulted in a greater reduction in mortality than annual clinical examination alone [51]. After 8 years of follow-up there was no difference in risk of breast cancer death in the 19 711 women randomised to mammography and clinical examination relative to the 19 694 women in the clinical examination alone group (RR 0.97, 95% CI 0.62–1.52). This trial has been criticised for lack of statistical power, for use of volunteers rather than a representative population, and for poor quality mammography especially in its early years [45]. But its result raises the important question of the extent to which clinical examination alone, despite its lower sensitivity, could reduce breast cancer mortality. This has never been tested in a randomised controlled trial but is a priority for future research, especially in developing counties with rising mortality from breast cancer but which do not have the resources for mammography screening.

Further evidence strengthening the conclusion that screening which includes mammography is effective in reducing breast cancer deaths comes from the UK Trial of Early Detection of Breast Cancer [80] which, after 10 years, found that two health districts in which all women aged 45–64 years had been offered screening by clinical examination and mammography had 20% fewer breast cancer deaths than comparison districts with no intervention (RR 0.80, 95% CI 0.69–0.94). Likewise case-control studies in Nijmegen [81], Utrecht [21] and Florence [61] which compared the risk of breast cancer death in screened versus unscreened women from the same population, found relative risks of 0.48, 0.30 and 0.53, respectively. However, as pointed out in Chapter 1, such studies are liable to selection bias, in that women at higher risk of breast cancer death are less likely to be screened, so that not all of the observed reduction in risk may be the result of screening [54]. The US Breast Cancer Detection Demonstration Project also studied self-selected women who had volunteered for screening; Morrison et al. [53] used all their known risk factors for breast cancer to construct a theoretical control population, and using US mortality rates estimated that women enrolled in the project had 20% fewer deaths than expected.

Effectiveness of Screening Younger Women

Although the effectiveness of mammographic screening in reducing mortality from breast cancer is generally considered proven for women aged 50 years or over when first screened, there remains considerable controversy about the effect of such screening in younger women. Some authors consider that there is sufficient evidence to support routine screening from age 40 years [48], whereas others suggest that any possible benefit is so small that even a randomised trial of screening at such ages is not justified [9].

Much of the disagreement is a result of the fact that, with the exception of the Canadian trial, none of the studies which have reported on mortality to date has been designed to demonstrate a benefit in specific age subgroups. In general, trials which have reported results for such subgroups have shown less benefit in the women below 50 years at age of entry, and in the HIP study the effect of screening in women aged 40–49 years took longer to become apparent [69]. After 18 years there was a relative risk of 0.76 (95% CI 0.50–1.16). In Stockholm, after 7 years of follow-up the relative risk was 1.07 (0.53–2.16) [34], and in the Swedish Two-County study after 8 years the relative risk was 0.92 (0.52, 1.60). For the UKTEDBC [80], however, women aged 45–49 years at entry had the largest benefit of any subgroup, although there were no significant differences between age groups. Screening also appears to be less sensitive in younger women [73] and a shorter screening interval may be required to achieve a mortality reduction. However, as observed above, the confidence intervals surrounding the estimated relative risks are wide. Overviews of a number of trials can overcome this problem to some extent, and the overview of various Swedish trials found a relative risk of 0.87 in women aged 40–49 years at entry, with 95% CI (0.63–1.20) [57]. However, such analyses are hampered by the fact that it is difficult to determine how much of the benefit was in fact due to repeated screening after age 50 years. In addition, one of the trials included only women aged 45 years and above, and found a much greater benefit in women aged 45–49 years at entry than in those aged 50–54 years [32].

The Canadian Trial

As described above, one arm of the Canadian National Breast Screening study was specifically designed to study the effect of screening by mammography in women aged 40–49 years [50]. However, the trial has been plagued by controversy for a period of years [45]. Part of the problem is that the sample size of the trial was inadequate, since no account was taken in the calculations of the restriction of breast cancer deaths to those in cases diagnosed after the start of the trial. Another problem has been caused by the use of a volunteer population, and the fact that women randomised to the control group had a baseline clinical examination, and were encouraged to perform breast self-examination, the effect of either of which on subsequent mortality is unknown.

The first mortality results showed, after 7 years, a relative risk of breast cancer death of 1.08 in the women allocated to the mammography arm, with 95% confidence interval 0.59–1.80 [50]. However, in addition to the problems described above, there has also been considerable debate about the quality of mammography in at least some of the centres participating in the trial, although this is disputed by the principal investigators [4]. Nevertheless, the contribution of these various factors means that the trial, at least at present, cannot resolve the question of whether screening younger women reduces their risk of breast cancer death.

The UK Trial

In 1990, a multicentre trial was begun in the UK, with the aim of estimating the benefit of starting mammography screening at ages 40 or 41 years compared with the effect of starting at age 50 as in the current UK national programme. The trial is intended to recruit 195 000 women aged 40–41 years at entry, two-thirds being randomised to a control group, with no intervention until they enter the national programme at age 50 years, and one-third to a study group offered annual screening by mammography. The trial is designed to show a 20% reduction in breast cancer mortality over 10 years in the group offered screening, with 80% power. A trial is currently being proposed in Europe with a broadly similar protocol which will enhance the probability of obtaining an answer to this important question.

Effectiveness of Breast Self-Examination

Many health educators actively encourage women to examine their own breasts regularly as a form of self-screening. But it is much more difficult to evaluate self-screening than an organised professional screening programme and, despite many studies, it is still not clear whether or not breast self-examination (BSE) can substantially reduce the risk of breast cancer death.

In the UK Trial of Early Detection of Breast Cancer, 63571 women aged 45–64 years in two health districts were sent a personal invitation to attend a class where they were taught, in groups, how to practice regular breast self-examination, what signs to look out for, and what to do if they suspected any abnormality. A self-referral diagnostic clinic was provided for their use. In one district, 53% of invited women attended the class, but in the other only 31% did so [78]. In the former district performance of BSE was assessed by interview in a random sample of 800 women before they were invited to a class and again one year later [17]. It was found that before the programme 24% of women were performing BSE at least monthly, and apparently using an appropriate technique. One year later the proportion doing so had increased to 41% overall ($p < 0.001$) but in the women who attended the class the proportion had increased from 28% before invitation to 47% one year later ($p < 0.001$). The validity of self-reported BSE practice could not be assessed but at least knowledge had been increased in those who attended the class. Over the ensuing 10 years breast cancer mortality in these two districts was compared with that in four comparison districts where no intervention had been offered. Taking the two BSE districts together there was no difference from the comparison districts in 10-year breast cancer mortality (RR 1.07 95% CI 0.93–1.22), suggesting that this public health education campaign had had no effect [30]. There was, however, a surprising difference between the two districts – that in which response to the teaching had been only 31%, having significantly lower breast cancer mortality than the district with the higher initial response. But since this trial was not randomised, a number of factors other than practice of BSE could have contributed to the difference, including different trends in underlying mortality, and different treatment policies [30].

Another large prospective study of BSE was undertaken in Finland by Gastrin et al. [35]. Women's clubs were invited to participate in a health education programme, consisting of initial classes given by health professionals, followed by regular encouragement by key lay volunteers, and the distribution of calendars to record practice of BSE, which were returned to a central office every 2 years. Out of 56177 women aged 20 years or over, 29018 (52%) returned calendars reporting monthly BSE and are regarded as compliers. After excluding women with pre-existing breast cancer and those with breast cancer diagnosed in the first two years (who may have been symptomatic at the start) the remaining cohort of 28785 women were followed for up to 14 years from date of enrollment. Their subsequent incidence of breast cancer was slightly higher than the national incidence (rate ratio 1.2) but the stage distribution as recorded in the Cancer Registry did not differ significantly from that for the whole of Finland in 1980 (the middle year of the follow-up study). However, their mortality from breast cancer did differ significantly from that expected in Finland, with a relative risk of 0.71 (95% CI 0.57–0.87). The all-cause mortality of this cohort was also lower, and their socioeconomic status slightly higher than national rates. Selection bias (both in those belonging to these clubs and in the 52% who were BSE compliers) cannot be ruled out as an explanation for their lower than expected risk of breast cancer death.

Selection bias may also affect retrospective case-control studies, although this did not appear to influence the results in a study within an American health maintenance organisation [56]. This compared self-reported BSE practice in the year prior to diagnosis in patients with advanced breast cancer (cases) with that up to a similar reference date in age-matched controls. After adjusting for various confounding variables (including use of professional screening) the relative risk of advanced breast cancer in BSE practitioners was 1.15 (95% CI 0.73–1.81). Cases and controls did not differ significantly in their frequency of BSE, but in the few women with high proficiency scores (judged by questionnaire) there did seem to be a reduction in risk of advanced disease. Overall, however, this paper concluded that BSE as practised by most women in their population is of little or no benefit.

Thus, although there may be a benefit to an individual woman who practises BSE assiduously and proficiently, it has so far proved impossible to demonstrate convincingly that a public health education programme results in lower mortality. Further trials using cluster randomisation are currently underway in Russia and in China.

Disadvantages and Costs of Breast Screening

The adverse health effects can be classified as those arising from the actual screening process, those arising from false positive results, and those arising from diagnosis of breast cancer.

Morbidity from the Screening Process

Since the early days of mammography screening, concern has been expressed about the induction of radiogenic breast cancers caused by exposing the breast to X-irradiation [3]. Retrospective studies of women who have received large doses of medical radiation, and studies of nuclear bomb survivors have confirmed an excess risk of breast cancer arising 10–20 years later. Extrapolating from the exposure data of these studies, the risks associated with exposure to the low doses of radiation given by modern mammography (mean absorbed dose of 0.5–3.0 mGy) have been estimated [36]. Among one million women screened once at age 50 years it is suggested that 21 extra cancers would arise in their lifetime, compared with an expected underlying lifetime incidence (in the United States) of about 80 000 per million. Making assumptions about the mortality rate and the proportion of deaths prevented by screening, the ratio of deaths avoided to cancers induced approaches 600 to 1. For women aged 40 years, however, the radiogenic risk is greater (78 new cancers per million women) and the benefit is unproven. Even though the balance of risk against benefit in those over 50 years is so small, it is highly desirable that mammographic screening units, as part of their quality assurance procedures, should routinely measure their radiation dose levels, and keep them down to the lowest level compatible with good image quality.

Induction of anxiety has also been postulated as an adverse consequence of encouraging women to attend for screening. It is suggested that heightening women's awareness of their vulnerability to breast cancer may cause them to worry excessively, and that psychological morbidity may be found both in those who accept screening and in those who reject it "because they would prefer not to know". However, psychological studies comparing women who have not been invited or encouraged to be screened with those attending a screening clinic found no significant difference in anxiety and stress levels [25]. Similarly no difference has been found in these respects between women who accept an invitation to be screened and those who do not [43].

Discomfort and pain caused by compression of the breast against the X-ray plate is a relatively minor disadvantage. One British study interviewed 597 women after they had been screened and reported that 35% of women experienced discomfort and 6% pain, which usually lasted less than 10 min [17, 68]. Other preventive procedures such as a dental filling or a cervical smear were considered to be more uncomfortable by a majority of women. Similar findings were reported by a US study of over 1800 women [71].

Morbidity Resulting from False Positive Results

As already seen, some breast cancer screening programmes have a relatively low specificity, referring 5% of women or more for investigation of suspicious screening test results, of whom only about one tenth turn out to have cancer. Using a combination of diagnostic tests including further mammographic views, clinical examination, ultrasound and fine needle aspiration cytology, the great majority of these false positive referrals can be diagnosed as non-malignant without recourse to diagnostic biopsy [19].

The anxiety caused to women who are told that they have to return for further tests because of a suspicious finding is a cause for concern, and there are many anecdotal reports of individual women who have been extremely worried. However, the few systematic investigations of anxiety and depression that have been conducted in these women are reassuring. Ellman et al. [29] compared levels of psychological morbidity in nearly 2000 women, one-third of whom were recalled from screening for further investigation, one-third had been referred for investigation because of symptoms, and, the remainder, serving as a control group, were women attending for routine screening. All completed a standard validated questionnaire while in the clinic waiting-room, which may be the time of maximum anxiety. Six patients whose investigation resulted in a diagnosis of cancer were excluded from the analysis. Of the remainder the most anxious group were the symptomatic patients, followed by the women referred because of a positive mammogram, with those attending for routine screening having lower levels; the only statistically significant difference was between the symptomatic group and the routine screening group. Three months later the same women were sent a postal questionnaire, the results of which showed that although the symptomatic group still had increased anxiety, there was no persistent excess anxiety in women referred from screening. Similarly another study found no persistent anxiety six weeks after referral for investigation nor in women who had had to undergo excision biopsy with a benign result [15].

Morbidity Resulting from Diagnosis of Breast Cancer

The psychological morbidity resulting from a diagnosis of breast cancer is well documented in studies of symptomatic patients. In the context of screening it is a price that has to be paid for the benefit likely to derive from early diagnosis. But of all screen-detected cancers probably only one-fifth result in lives saved by screening [74], the remainder either being relatively slow-growing and curable even if left until symptomatic presentation, or being already incurable. It is in the group of slow-growing tumours that advancing the date of diagnosis may cause most harm, both psychological in that the woman and her family have to live longer with the permanent worry of breast cancer, and social in that it may affect her ability to obtain life insurance, mortgage cover, etc.

As with other screen-detected cancers, the possibility of overdiagnosis poses a particular problem. In the original screening trial in New York, the intervention group was no longer offered screening after the third round, and within 2 or 3 years the cumulative number of breast cancers diagnosed in the control group equalled that in the intervention group, indicating that there had been no overdiagnosis [69]. But with modern mammography, detection rates are higher, especially for ductal carcinoma in situ whose natural history is uncertain. In Nijmegen, 11% more cancers were found initially in a screened population than in geographic controls, but 8–12 years later the cumulative breast cancer rate in the controls had caught up, suggesting that the extra cancers diagnosed by screening would have presented symptomatically several years later [63]. In all subsequent trials, the control groups have also now been invited for screening. However, in the Swedish Two-County trial, it was noted that the cumulative control group incidence up to the date of their first invitation equalled that in the intervention group, after excluding prevalent cancers detected at the first screen [75]. It is, therefore, postulated that over-diagnosis is limited to cases diagnosed at the first screen, and also that it is concentrated in women below 50 years. In the Two-County trial, there were very few in situ cancers diagnosed after the first screen, but in the current UK breast screening programme, there has been no reduction in in situ rates in repeat rounds of screening [19].

Costs

Several studies have examined the resource costs of breast cancer screening. Obviously costs very enormously between different countries, not merely in currency rates, but for reasons connected with the organisation of health care, including the method and amount of payment for the many professionals involved. Hence comparisons of cost estimates between different countries are difficult to interpret.

A detailed costing of screening in Edinburgh was conducted in the mid-1980s [20]. This examined in detail the unit costs of mammography clinical examination, cytology and biopsy and took into account the costs of recruitment, capital costs for equipment, etc, and overhead costs. Updated to 1992/93, this resulted in an estimate (including the costs of assessment of women referred) of £22.60 per woman screened, or £4300 per cancer detected [personal communication]. A similar exercise in Australia [44] in 1994 found a cost of $A 117.70 per woman screened, and $A 11 550 per cancer detected.

These estimates need to be set against the benefit in terms of lives saved or life-years gained in order to assess the cost-effectiveness of screening. Putting together the original costs from Edinburgh and the mortality reductions for women over 50 years found in the Two-County and HIP trials, Forrest et al. [33] calculated that a 3-yearly mammographic screening programme would cost £3500 (1986 prices) for each year of life saved.

Conclusions

Screening postmenopausal women for breast cancer using mammography can reduce their risk of dying from breast cancer. In a population of women aged 50–74 years at least 70% of whom accept screening, regular mammography at intervals no longer than 3 years can reduce breast cancer mortality by 20%–25%. Apart from resource costs, the disadvantages imposed by screening women in this age-group are judged by most authorities to be acceptably small in relation to the benefit. For premenopausal women, however, the size of any mortality reduction has not yet been quantified and may be less than in older age-groups because screening is probably less sensitive at detecting cancer in premenopausal breasts. Clinical examination is a less sensitive test than mammography and its effectiveness in reducing mortality in any age-group has not been tested. Similarly the effect of education in breast self-examination has not yet been convincingly demonstrated, a major problem being the difficulty of persuading sufficient women to practise it with a high level of proficiency. Randomised controlled trials addressing these unresolved issues are starting in several countries, but are unlikely to reach conclusions for at least 10 years.

References

1. Alexander FE, Anderson TJ, Brown HK et al. (1994) The Edinburgh randomised trial of breast cancer screening: results after 10 years of follow-up. Br J Cancer 70:542–548.
2. Andersson I, Aspergren K, Janzon L et al. (1988) Mammographic screening and mortality from breast cancer: the Malmo mammographic screening trial. Br Med J 297:943–948.
3. Bailar JC (1976) Mammography: a contrary view. Ann Intern Med 84:77–84.

4. Baines CJ (1994) The Canadian National Breast Screening Study: a perspective on criticisms. Ann Intern Med 120:326–334.
5. Baines CJ, Miller AB, Bassett AA et al. (1989) Physical examination: evaluation of its role as a single screening modality in the Canadian National Breast Screening Study. Cancer 63:160–166.
6. Baker L (1982) Breast Cancer Detection Demonstration Project: five year summary report. CA 32:194–225.
7. Beck JS and Members of the MRC Breast Tumour Pathology Panel (1985) Observer variability in reporting of breast lesions. J Clin Pathol 38:1358–1365.
8. Beral V, Hermon L, Reeves G, Peto R (1995) Sudden fall in breast cancer death (letter) rates in England and Wales. Lancet 345:1642–1643
9. Beral V (1993) Breast cancer – mammographic screening. Lancet 341:1509–1510.
10. Bernstein L, Ross RK (1993) Endogenous hormones and breast cancer risk. Epidemiol Rev 15:48–65.
11. Berrino F, Panico S, Muti P (1989) Dietary fat, nutritional status and endocrine-associated cancers. In: Miller AB (ed) Diet and the aetiology of cancer. Springer-Verlag, Berlin, pp 3–12.
12. Berrino F, Sant M, Verdecchia et al. (1995) Survival of cancer patients in Europe. IARC Scientific Publications, no. 32, Lyon.
13. Black RJ, Sharp L, Kendrick SW (1993) Trends in cancer survival in Scotland, 1968–1990. Information and Statistics Division, ISD Publications, Edinburgh.
14. Brown J, Rodway A, Chamberlain J et al. (1994) The effect of fine needle aspiration cytology on the number of diagnostic biopsies and time to diagnosis in a breast screening programme. Breast 3:103–108.
15. Bull AR, Campbell MJ (1994). Assessment of the psychological impact of a breast screening programme. Br J Radiol 64:510–515.
16. Bush TL, Helzlsouer KJ (1993) Tamoxifen for the primary prevention of breast cancer: a review and critique of the concept and trial. Epidemiol Rev 15:233–243.
17. Calnan MW, Chamberlain J, Moss S (1984) Compliance with a class teaching breast self examination. J Epidemiol Commun Health 37:264–270.
18. Cancer Research Campaign (1989) Factsheet 6.2.
19. Chamberlain J, Moss SM, Kirkpatrick AE, Michell M, Johns L (1993) National Health Service breast screening programme results for 1991–2. Br Med J 307:353–356.
20. Clarke PR, Fraser NM (1991) Economic analysis of screening for breast cancer. Report for Scottish Home and Health Department, Edinburgh.
21. Collette HJA, Day NE, Rombach JJ, de Waard F (1984) Evaluation of screening for breast cancer in a non-randomised study (the DOM Project) by means of a case-control study. Lancet i:1224–1225.
22. Darby SC, Doll R, Gill SK et al. (1987) Long term mortality after a simple treatment course with x-rays in patients treated for ankylosing spondylitis. Br J Cancer 55:179–190.
23. de Waard T, de Loive JWJ, Baanders-Van Halewijn EA (1960) On the bimodal age distribution of mammary carcinoma. Br J Cancer 14:437–448.
24. de Waard F, Trichopoulos D (1988) A unifying concept of the aetiology of breast cancer. Int J Cancer 41:666–669.
25. Dean C, Roberts MM, French K, Robinson S (1986) Psychiatric morbidity after screening for breast cancer. J Epidemiol Community Health 40:71–75.
26. Dupont WD, Page DL (1985) Risk factors for breast cancer in women with proliferative breast disease. N Engl J Med 312:146–151.

27. Dupont WD, Page DL, Parl FF et al. (1994) Long-term risk of breast cancer in women with fibroadenoma. N Engl J Med 331:10–15.
28. Early Breast Cancer Trialists' Collaborative Group (1992) Systemic treatment of early breast cancer by hormonal, cytotoxic, or immune therapy. Lancet 339:1–15.
29. Ellman R, Angeli N, Christians A, Moss S, Chamberlain J, Maguire P (1989) Psychiatric morbidity associated with screening for breast cancer. Br J Cancer 60:781–784.
30. Ellman R, Moss SM, Coleman D, Chamberlain J (1993) Breast self-examination programmes in the trial of early detection of breast cancer: ten year findings. Br J Cancer 68:208–212.
31. Feuer EJ, Wun L-M (1992) How much of the recent rise in breast cancer incidence can be explained by increases in mammography utilization? Am J Epidemiol 136:1423–1436.
32. Fletcher SW, Black W, Harris R, Rimer BK, Shapiro S (1993) Report of the International Workshop on Screening for Breast Cancer. J Natl Cancer Inst 85:1645–1656.
33. Forrest APM (1986) Breast cancer screening report to the health ministers of England, Wales, Scotland and Northern Ireland. London: HMSO.
34. Frisell J, Eklund G, Hellstrom L, Lidbrink E, Rutqvist LE, Somell A (1991) Randomized study of mammography screening – preliminary report on mortality in the Stockholm trial. Breast Cancer Res Treat 18:49–56.
35. Gastrin G, Miller AB, To T et al. (1994) Incidence and mortality from breast cancer in the Mama Program for breast screening in Finland, 1973–1986. Cancer 73:2168–2174.
36. Gohagen JK, Darby WP, Spitznagal EL, Monsees BS, Tome AE (1986) Radiogenic breast cancer effects of mammographic screening. J Natl Cancer Inst 77:71–76.
37. Goodwin PJ, Boyd NF (1988) Mammographic parenchymal pattern and breast cancer risk: a critical appraisal of the evidence. Am J Epidemiol 127:1097–1108
38. Greenwald P, Kramer B, Weed D (1993) Expanding horizons in breast and prostate cancer prevention and early detection. J Cancer Educ 8:91–107.
39. Guyer PB (1993) Breast ultrasound. In: Tucker A (ed) Textbook of Mammography. Churchill Livingstone, Edinburgh, pp 211–243.
40. Haybittle J (1991) Curability of breast cancer. Br Med Bull 47:319–323.
41. Hoffman DA, Lonstein JE, Morin MM et al. (1989) Breast cancer in women with scoliosis exposed to multiple diagnostic x-rays. J Natl Cancer Inst 81:1307–1312.
42. Houlston RS, McCarter E, Parbhoo S, Scurr JH, Slack J (1992) Family history and risk of breast cancer. J Med Genet 29:154–157.
43. Hunt SM, Alexander F, Roberts M (1988) Attenders and non-attenders at a breast screening clinic: a comparative study. Public Health 102:3–10.
44. Hurley SF, Livingstone PM, Thane N, Quang L (1994) Mammographic screening: measurement of the cost in a population based programme in Victoria, Australia. J Epidemiol Comm Health 48:391–399.
45. Kopans DB, Feig SA (1993) The Canadian National Breast Screening Study: a critical review. AJR 161:755–760.
46. Koscielny S, Le MG, Tubiana M (1989) The natural history of human breast cancer. The relationship between involvement of axillary lymph nodes and the initiation of distant metastases. Br J Cancer 59:775–782.
47. Lloyd Williams K, Phillips PH, Jones PA, Beaman SA, Fleming PJ (1990) Thermography for screening for breast cancer. J Epidemiol Comm Health 44(2):112–113.
48. Mettlin C, Smart CR (1994) Breast cancer detection guidelines for women aged 40 to 49 years: rationale for the American Cancer Society Reaffirmation of recommenda-

tions. CA 44:248–255.

49. Miki Y, Swensen J, Shattuck-Eidens D et al. (1994) A strong candidate for the breast and ovarian cancer susceptibility gene BRCA1. Science 266:66–71.

50. Miller AB, Baines CJ, To T, Wall C (1992) Canadian National Breast Screening Study: 1. Breast cancer detection and death rates among women aged 40 to 49 years. Can Med Assoc J 147:1459–1476.

51. Miller AB, Baines CJ, To T, Wall C (1992) Canadian National Breast Screening Study: 2. Breast cancer detection and death rates among women aged 50 to 59 years. Can Med Assoc J 147:1477–1488.

52. Mittra I (1994) Breast screening: the case for physical examination without mammography. Lancet 343:342–344.

53. Morrison AS, Brisson J, Khalid N (1988) Breast cancer incidence and mortality in the Breast Cancer Detection Demonstration Project. J Natl Cancer Inst 80:1540–1547.

54. Moss SM, Summerley ME, Thomas BT, Ellman R, Chamberlain J (1992) A case-control evaluation of the effect of breast cancer screening in the United Kingdom trial of early detection of breast cancer. J Epidemiol Comm Health 46:362–364.

55. Moss SM, Coleman DA, Ellman R et al. (1993) Interval cancers and sensitivity in the screening centres of the UK Trial of Early Detection of Breast Cancer. Eur J Cancer 29A:225–258.

56. Newcomb PA, Weiss NS, Storer BE, Scholes D, Young BE, Voigt LF (1991) Breast self-examination in relation to the occurrence of advanced breast cancer. J Natl Cancer Inst 83:260–265.

57. Nystrom L, Rutqvist LE, Wall S, et al. (1993) Breast cancer screening with mammography: overiview of Swedish randomised trials. Lancet 341:973–978.

58. Office of Population Censuses and Surveys (1993). 1992 Mortality statistics cause. HMSO, London.

59. Office of Population Censuses and Surveys (1993) 1987 Cancer statistics registrations. Series MB1, no. 20. HMSO, London.

60. Page DL, Dupont WD, Rogers LW, Landerberger M (1982) Intraductal carcinoma of the breast: follow-up after biopsy only. Cancer 49:751–758.

61. Palli D, del Turco MR, Buiatti E et al. (1986) A case-control study of the efficacy of a non-randomized breast cancer screening program in Florence (Italy). Int J Cancer 38:501–504.

62. Parkin DM, Pisani P, Ferlay J (1993) Estimates of the worldwide incidence of eighteen major cancer screening programmes. Br J Cancer 51:551–568.

63. Peeters PH, Verbeek AL, Straatman H et al. (1989) Evaluation of overdiagnosis of breast cancer in screening with mammography: results of the Nijmegen Programme. Int J Epidemiol 28:295–299.

64. Peeters PHM, Verbeek ALM, Hendriks JHCL et al. (1989) The occurrence of interval cancers in the Nijmegen screening programme. Br J Cancer 59:929–932.

65. Pike MC, Spicer DV, Dahmoush L, Press MF (1993) Estrogens, progestogens, normal breast cell proliferation and breast cancer risk. Epidemiol Rev 15:17–25.

66. Pisani P, Parkin DM, Ferlay J (1993) Estimates of the worldwide mortality from eighteen major cancers in 1985. Implications for prevention and projections of future burden. Int J Cancer 55:891–903.

67. Pocock S (1982) Long term survival analysis: the curability of breast cancer. Stats in Med 1:93–104.

68. Rutter DR, Calnan M, Vaile MSB, Field S, Wade KA (1992). Discomfort and pain during mammography: description, prediction and prevention. Br Med J 305:443–445.

69. Shapiro S, Venet W, Strax P, Venet L (1988) Periodic screening for breast cancer. In: The Health Insurance Plan Project and its sequelae, 1963–1986. Johns Hopkins University Press, Baltimore, London.

70. Spicer DV, Ursin G, Parisky YR et al. (1995). Changes in mammographic densities induced by a hormonal contraceptive designed to reduce breast cancer risk. J Natl Cancer Inst 86:431–436.

71. Stomper PC, Kopans DB, Sadowsky NL et al. (1988). Is mammography painful? A multicentre patient survey. Arch Intern Med 148:521–524.

72. Swift M, Morell D, Massey RB, Chase CL (1991) Incidence of cancer in 161 families affected by ataxis telangiectasia. N Engl J Med 325:1831–1836.

73. Tabar L, Fagerberg G, Day NE, Holmberg L (1987) What is the optimum interval between mammographic screening examinations? Br J Cancer 155:547–551.

74. Tabar L, Fagerberg G, Duffy SW, Day NE (1989) The Swedish two county trial of mammographic screening for breast cancer: recent results and calculation of benefit. J Epidemiol Community Health 43:107–114.

75. Tabar L, Fagerberg G, Duffy SW, Day NE, Gad A, Grontoft O (1992) Update of the Swedish two-county program of mammographic screening for breast cancer. Radiol Clin N Amer 30(1):187–210.

76. Tokanaga M, Land CE, Yamamoto T et al. (1987) Incidence of female breast cancer among atomic bomb survivors, Hiroshima and Nagasaki, 1950–1980. Radiat Res 112:243–272.

77. UK National Case-Control Study Group (1990) Oral contraceptive use and breast cancer in young women: subgroup anlayses. Lancet 335:1507–1509.

78. UK Trial of Early Detection of Breast Cancer Group (1981) Trial of early detection of breast cancer: description of method. Br J Cancer 44:618–627.

79. UK Trial of Early Detection of Breast Cancer Group (1992) Specificity of screening in United Kingdom trial of early detection of breast cancer. Br Med J 304:346–349.

80. UK Trial of Early Detection of Breast Cancer Group (1993) Breast cancer mortality after 10 years in the UK trial of early detection of breast cancer. Breast 2:13–20.

81. Verbeek ALM, Hendricks JHCL, Holland R, Mravunac M, Sturmans F, Day NE (1984) Reduction in breast cancer mortality through mass screening with modern mammography (first results of the Nijmegen Project 1975–81). Lancet i:1222–1224.

82. Wald NJ, Chamberlain J, Hackshaw A (1994) European Society of Mastology Consensus Conference on Breast Cancer Screening, Paris, 4–5 February 1993. Report of the Evaluation Committee. Clin Oncology 4:261–268.

83. Wolfe JN (1976) Risk for breast cancer development determined by mammographic parenchymal pattern. Cancer 37:2486–2492.

84. Wooster R, Neuhausen SL, Mangion J et al. (1994) Localization of a breast cancer susceptibility gene, BRCA2, to chromosome 13q12–13. Science 265:2088–2090.

85. Wright CJ (1986) Breast cancer screening: a different look at the evidence. Surgery 100:594–598.

4 – Screening for Colorectal cancer

Jocelyn Chamberlain

Introduction

Carcinoma of the large bowel is a common condition in developed countries accounting for 12% of cancer registrations and of cancer deaths in England and Wales. In both sexes it is the third commonest cause of cancer death, after lung and prostate cancer in men, and breast and lung cancer in women. In 1992, 8749 men and 8654 women died from colorectal cancer [44, 45].

Both incidence and mortality increase with increasing age, the disease becoming relatively frequent from about age 50 years onwards. The few cases at younger ages are often in people with one of the inherited risk syndromes discussed further below. The main impact of the disease is in people of retirement age, with 65% of new registrations and 79% of deaths occurring among people over the age of 65 years.

Of large bowel cancers, 40% occur in the rectum, 32% in the descending colon, 10% in the transverse colon (including flexures) and 18% in the ascending colon and caecum. Women have a slightly lower incidence of colon cancers than men at all ages, and rectal cancers increase with age more steeply in men so that the rate of rectal cancer in men in their seventies (110 per 100000) is twice that of women in their seventies (55 per 100000). There has been an increased incidence of right-sided colon cancers over the past few decades [1] so that the percentage distribution of colorectal tumour sites has shifted to the right [27].

Time Trends

Mortality from colorectal cancer in England and Wales has been falling over the past 40 years. Case fatality rates have improved only slowly over this time period and screening has not been practised, except in the small number of people with inherited risk. Therefore, most of the decline in mortality is probably attributable to a decline in incidence reflecting reduced exposure to aetiological agents.

National incidence rates for England and Wales are only available for the last 20 years and in most age-groups show an increasing incidence [45], which conflicts with the hypothesis that the fall in mortality is caused by lower risk of developing the disease. However, over this time period, Regional Cancer Registries have been improving their efficiency in ascertainment of cases, and this provides an explanation for a spurious increased incidence. In people below 60 years, registration rates have been falling implying that the reduction in incidence at younger ages more than compensates for the improved efficiency of registration. This suggests a cohort effect and cohort analyses of mortality do indeed confirm a decline in women born since 1930, and, for colon but not rectal cancer, for men born since 1950 [46].

Geographical Variation

There are major differences in the incidence of colorectal cancer across the world. Risk is highest in Australasia, North America and Northern Europe, and lowest in Africa and Asia, particularly India. Migrant studies, such as those in Japanese who have emigrated to the USA, show that within one or two generations the migrants' risk starts to approach that of the host population, providing strong support for an environmental aetiology [3].

Aetiology and Primary Prevention

Diet is the most obvious environmental agent and various components of diet have been implicated as either protective or causative agents. Noting the low incidence of colorectal cancer in African Blacks compared to Europeans, Burkitt [8] proposed that a high fibre diet was protective, acting by increasing faecal bulk and reducing transit time through the large bowel. This hypothesis has been extensively researched by comparing past dietary fibre intake in patients with colorectal cancer and controls, and in a few prospective studies [6]. The active ingredient of fibre is now recognised to be non-starch polysaccharides which are predominant in fruit and vegetables and also in bran. Most human studies have found no protective effect from cereal consumption, but have found a reduced risk associated with high consumption of fruit and vegetables. One hypothesis is that non-starch polysaccharides act as an energy substrate for colonic bacteria thus promoting fermentation which in turn leads to dilution of faecal mass, shorter transit time, and reduction of faecal mutagenicity [6]. It is also possible that starch may be protective although this is still uncertain.

Dietary fat has been implicated as a causative agent, although it is uncertain whether its role is merely a reflection of total calorie intake, or of specific fatty acids. Ecological comparisons of colorectal cancer incidence in different countries and national consumption figures for the same countries suggest that animal fat is more important. From studies of the role of bile acids, Hill [21] postulates that fatty acids are important as promoters of carcinogenesis in colorectal adenomas, but not as initiators of adenoma formation.

Other aetiological dietary factors include alcohol, although it is not known whether the positive associations which have been found are due to alcohol itself or to its calorie content; and coffee, which appears to be protective, although not due to its caffeine content.

It is unlikely that experimental randomised controlled trials of dietary change on a whole population basis will ever be done on a sufficient scale to demonstrate the extent of any reduction in colorectal cancer which could be achieved. Nevertheless in the light of current knowledge it is reasonable to advocate a diet high in non-starch polysaccharides and low in fat, particularly animal fat. Such a "prudent" diet is of course also relevant for protection against cardiovascular disease.

The change to greater consumption of fibre-containing foods and lower consumption of saturated fats that has occurred in the UK within the last decade cannot, however, explain the falling incidence of colorectal cancer which started in younger people 20 years ago; this may have been associated with increasing fresh fruit and vegetable consumption. The effect of more recent changes in dietary fashion is as yet unclear and is likely to take several years to work through to a reduced incidence.

High-Risk Groups for Colorectal Cancer

Although the great majority of colorectal cancers have an environmental aetiology, an important subgroup with a genetic susceptibility to colorectal cancer exists. As with other inherited cancer risks, subjects in these families tend to develop their cancer at a much earlier age. Recognised syndromes include familial adenomatous polyposis and hereditary non-polyposis colorectal cancer. These families have proved to be the starting point for identification of genetic abnormalities some of which, e.g. APC, are also present in sporadic colorectal cancer. Further families, with one or more affected relatives, may be at risk because of a combination of inherited and environmental factors, and in total, familial colorectal cancers may comprise up to 20% of all colorectal cancers. Depending on their level of risk, which can now be more precisely defined, current management of patients at familial risk ranges from total colectomy to regular endoscopic surveillance, with or without faecal occult blood testing. Another group at high risk of colorectal cancer are patients with ulcerative colitis.

Natural History

It is known from histopathology studies that some colorectal carcinomas develop in adenomatous polyps, and this "adenoma–carcinoma sequence" [40] is widely accepted as being the principal source of carcinomas, apart from those associated with ulcerative colitis. Polyps in the large bowel may be hyperplastic or adenomatous, only the latter having the potential to become malignant. This adenoma–carcinoma natural history is clearly very relevant to screening, since if it were possible to detect and remove premalignant adenomas, the incidence of subsequent carcinoma would fall. But for this, we need to know the proportion of adenomas which progress to carcinoma, the distribution of their progression over time, and the proportion of cancers which do not go through a detectable adenomatous phase.

The prevalence of adenomas at autopsy has been studied in several countries, the differences between them mirroring international differences in colorectal cancer incidence. Within the UK, two studies [10, 68] found a prevalence of adenoma in men who had died of causes other than colorectal cancer of 37%–39% and in women of 29%–30%. Prevalence increased with increasing age, rising to 40%–60% in people over 75 years. The cumulative incidence of colorectal cancer up to age 74 years is only about 4% and to 84 years, 12% [39]. Therefore it is clear that the great majority of adenomas do not progress.

Histopathology studies have found that the malignant potential of an adenoma is directly related to its size, to whether it has a tubular (good prognosis) or villous (poor prognosis) histology and to the degree of dysplasia. This implies either a progression of epithelial changes of increasing severity as the adenoma grows over time, or that only high-risk adenomas have the potential for growth.

The fact that some of the genetic mutations identified in colorectal cancers are also present in adenomas adds weight to the theory of the adenoma–carcinoma sequence [64]. Studies in vitro, using a human colonic adenoma cell line with a K-*ras* gene mutation, have found that it can undergo spontaneous malignant transformation, becoming less responsive to the growth-inhibiting effects of transforming growth factor beta. Moreover chromosomal changes, involving chromosome 18 (containing the putative tumour suppressor gene DCC, deleted in colon cancer) accompany the malignant transformation [36]. Multiple mutations in oncogenes and tumour suppressor genes seem to underlie the malignant transformation.

Very few studies have followed-up diagnosed adenomatous polyps without treatment by excision, a situation which has become even more unusual with the advent of flexible sigmoidoscopy and colonoscopy. Stryker et al. [60] undertook a follow-up of 2226 patients who had had adenomas with diameter of 1 cm or greater, diagnosed radiologically. Using a lifetable analysis they found that within 5 years of diagnosis 2.5% of patients had developed colorectal cancer, within 10 years 8% and within 20 years 24%. In a study of 215 polyps measuring less than 5 mm, Hoff et al. [23] noted that of 35 adenomas, 17 increased in size over a 2-year period, 13 remained unchanged and five became smaller, suggesting that regression may also be possible. Eide [15] modelled the risk of development of cancer from data on the age-specific autopsy prevalence of adenomas and the cumulative incidence of carcinoma in Norway. He estimated that if *all* the carcinomas developed from adenomas the annual rate of conversion from adenoma into carcinoma was 0.25%. If all the carcinomas arose from adenomas greater than 1 cm in diameter the annual conversion rate would be 3%. Similar estimates for villous adenomas and those with severe dysplasia were 17% and 37%, respectively.

There is histopathological evidence suggesting that up to 40% of cancers do *not* go through a detectable premalignant adenomatous phase. There are theoretical reasons to suppose that such cancers are more rapidly progressive and, therefore, more likely to cause death. Adenoma remnants are found less often in poorly differentiated cancers [14], and an inverse relationship has been shown between the stage of carcinoma and the number of synchronous polyps [53]. It is, therefore, important that screening to detect adenomas should be judged not only in terms of its effectiveness in reducing incidence but also in its long-term effectiveness in reducing mortality.

Prognosis of Colorectal Carcinomas

As with other tumours, prognosis varies according to stage at diagnosis. Dukes' classification of stage, used internationally, subdivides carcinomas according to their degree of local invasion. Stage A is confined within the bowel wall, Stage B has penetrated the bowel wall, and Stage C has local lymph node involvement. An even more advanced degree of disease, with liver metastases, is often called Stage D.

The prognosis for Stage A tumours is very good, with a 5-year survival of over 80%, falling to 58% for Stage B, 27% for Stage C and less than 10% for Stage D [59]. Clinical series commonly report less than 10% of patients presenting at Stage A, and over half presenting with Stage C or D tumours.

There are few reports of population-based stage-distribution or stage-specific incidence rates, but randomised controlled trials of screening (described in detail below) provide one source. In the large Nottingham trial [20] among a control unscreened population of 53 885 people aged 45–74 years, 123 cancers were found in the first three years. Thirteen (11%) were Stage A, 40 (32%) Stage B, 40 (32%) Stage C, and 26 (21%) Stage D. Four were unstaged. With longer follow-up in this study it has been noted that in this same unscreened population there has been a significant shift to an earlier stage distribution within rectal cancers from 9.9% to 27.5% Stage A, but no change of stage distribution of colon cancers [49]. This is attributed to increasing awareness of the symptoms of rectal cancer among general practitioners participating in the trial.

Overall Survival

Overall 5-year survival has shown a small but steady improvement over time. In Scotland for example [7], 5-year relative survival improved from 33.1% in cases diagnosed in 1968–72, to 39.6% in cases diagnosed in 1983–87. These trends probably reflect improvements in diagnostic and therapeutic management over time and this can be expected to continue with accumulating evidence that adjuvant chemotherapy (5-fluorouracil and levamisole) for patients with Stage B and C reduces case-fatality [13]. Further trials, including the use of adjuvant radiotherapy, are in progress.

The Rationale for Screening

The trends of decreasing incidence and improving survival offer hope that colorectal cancer may not be such a large problem in the future as it is today. However, the dietary or other changes contributing to reduced incidence have a long latent interval before their contributions may be fully seen, and the improvements in survival are small and limited to certain subgroups of patients. Therefore, for the foreseeable future, screening is a potentially more effective means of control.

The adenoma–carcinoma sequence on one hand, and the excellent survival of patients diagnosed with a Stage A tumour on the other suggest that screening could be a two-pronged weapon. Detection and removal of premalignant adenomas could prevent the development of cancers and thus reduce incidence, and, to an extent yet to be determined, mortality. Detection of invasive cancers at an earlier stage could result in a greater proportion being cured, and thus also reduce mortality.

Screening Methods

Endoscopic Screening

Rigid sigmoidoscopy, and more recently fibreoptic flexible sigmoidoscopy, have been used in general population screening. Colonoscopy, because of its greater complexity including the need for sedation, is not suitable as a general screening test but may be used in individuals at high risk including surveillance of patients who have had a previous adenoma.

The sensitivity of sigmoidoscopic methods for detecting both cancers and adenomas in theory could be 100% for neoplasia within the range of the instrument – 25 cm for rigid and 60 cm for flexible sigmoidoscopy. In practice, insertion to the fullest depth is not possible in a proportion of subjects, and other factors such as inadequate bowel preparation limit sensitivity further. Maule [38], in a study of 2611 patients, noted that flexible sigmoidoscopy reached 60 cm in only 39% of men and 17% of women. One Dukes' A carcinoma was found 16 months after a negative sigmoidoscopy. A case-control study of the efficacy of screening [55] reported that 11 cases of rectal carcinoma which subsequently led to death, were diagnosed within 3 years of a negative sigmoidoscopy. The denominator for estimating sensitivity as a proportion was not available from this study. Clearly neoplasia proximal to the depth of insertion cannot be detected. In practice, therefore, rigid sigmoidoscopy can detect at most 30%–40% of colorectal neoplasia and flexible sigmoidoscopy 60%–70%.

It is not appropriate to use the occurrence of interval cancers following endoscopy screening to derive a measure of sensitivity for cancer detection using the proportional incidence method, because the same screening test can also identify adenomas whose removal should reduce the subsequent incidence of cancer. Similarly it is not appropriate to use the occurrence of interval adenomas because the great majority of adenomas are asymptomatic and any that are diagnosed will not represent the total number that may be present. The occurrence of cancers following adenoma removal is discussed further below in the section on effectiveness of screening.

The specificity of sigmoidoscopy depends on the definition of a false positive. False positive results for cancer are not discussed in the literature on sigmoidoscopic screening but as far as detection of adenomas is concerned, non-adenomatous hyperplastic polyps can be regarded as false positives. Some argue that tubular adenomas less than 1 cm (approximately half of all adenomas) carry no excess risk of subsequent cancer [4], in which case they too could be regarded as false positives. In order to diagnose whether a polyp is a true or a false positive it is necessary to remove it and examine it histologically. The polyp(s) can be removed during sigmoidoscopy, possibly at the same time as the screening examination. Since most studies do not report on their hyperplastic polyps it is not possible to derive a quantitative estimate of specificity or positive predictive value.

Faecal Occult Blood Tests

The premise underlying the use of faecal occult blood tests (FOBTs) for screening, is that asymptomatic colorectal cancers and large adenomas bleed. But it is known that bleeding from colonic neoplasms is intermittent and that there is overlap with the volume of blood that is physiologically shed in the gut [2, 12]. Because of the intermittent nature of bleeding, FOBTs require that samples from several separate bowel motions should be tested in order to improve sensitivity. The generally accepted management of subjects with a positive FOBT is colonoscopy, and, in order to minimise the number of subjects undergoing this investigation, it is also important that the tests should have high specificity.

Many studies have examined the validity of different faecal occult blood tests in symptomatic patients who were in any case going to have colonoscopy. This enables a direct measure of sensitivity and specificity since the FOBT result can be compared with the "gold standard" findings at colonoscopy. However, the results in such subjects are not necessarily applicable to asymptomatic people undergoing screening.

The commonest FOBT which is being evaluated in several screening studies is Haemoccult II, a guaiac-based test which detects the pseudo-peroxidase activity of the heme component of haemoglobin. Subjects are provided with a kit of three test cards, each with two windows containing guaiac-impregnated filter paper. Subjects are instructed to collect their stool on three consecutive days using a paper sling across the lavatory bowl. Using one of the spatulas provided in the kit they take a small (pea-size) sample of each stool and place it on one of the windows, then repeat this from another area of the stool and place it on the second window. The test card is then sealed, and when all 3 have been completed, is taken or mailed back to the screening centre. Here a drop of hydrogen peroxide is applied to the reverse side of each of the six windows; a blue colour appearing at 30 seconds indicates a positive test.

Peroxidase-rich vegetables and red meat can give positive results. For this reason dietary restriction for two to three days before the test is sometimes recommended in order to reduce false positives. Similarly, subjects are asked to avoid taking nonsteroidal anti-inflammatory drugs prior to the test to minimise the likelihood of a false positive result from upper gastrointestinal bleeding.

The sensitivity of Haemoccult II has been studied in patients with known cancers and adenomas, comparing its results with the true situation found at colonoscopy. In one such study performed under carefully standardised conditions [52] the test was positive in 95 out of 107 patients with cancer (sensitivity 89%) but in only 19 out of 45 patients with adenomas larger than 1 cm (sensitivity 42%). Similar earlier studies had found lower levels of sensitivity in symptomatic neoplasia [12, 34]. In asymptomatic patients undergoing routine colonoscopy surveillance because of high risk, sensitivity has been found to be only 33% for cancers and 18%–24% for adenomas [51, 25].

In screening asymptomatic average-risk subjects by Haemoccult II, it is clearly unethical to subject those with negative results to colonoscopy so the true number of cancers present at the time of screening is unknown. As for other cancer sites, interval cancers presenting after a negative test are taken to be equivalent to false negatives. In one large study 76 cancers were found on screening 27 651 individuals and 20 interval cancers subsequently presented in people with negative Haemoccult results [20]. Using the conventional method of expressing sensitivity (screen-detected cancers divided by the sum of screen-detected and interval cancers) this gives a sensitivity of 78%, similar to the figure of 80.5% reported from Denmark [30]. Mandel et al. [35] reported a sensitivity of 80.8% in a trial involving 46 551 persons randomly allocated to annual FOBT, biennial FOBT or a control group. One way in which sensitivity can be increased is to rehydrate the Haemoccult filter-papers before testing. In Mandel's study this improved sensitivity to 92.2%. Kewenter et al. [28] in Sweden found that with unrehydrated specimens sensitivity was as low as 22%. Another method of improving sensitivity is to extend the testing period from 3 days to 6 days (giving 12 filter-papers for testing). This was shown to increase the yield of cancer in symptomatic patients [16] but gave only a small increased yield in asymptomatic subjects, most of which was offset by lower compliance with 6 day testing [61].

By using the proportional incidence method (Chapter 1) the estimate of sensitivity is considerably lower. This method, which can only be done in the context of a randomised controlled trial, provides an estimate of the proportion of cancers whose diagnosis was advanced by screening, in successive years after each screen. The number of cancers expected to arise in each year can be derived from the control group incidence, and by subtracting the number of interval cancers from this, the number of screen-detected cancers which would otherwise have presented in that year can be deduced, and expressed as a proportion of the total incidence. In the Nottingham trial of unrehydrated Haemoccult screening with a 2-year interval between screens, the sensitivity of screening was 59.5% for the first 12 months, falling to 54.1% for the period 12–24 months after screening (Moss et al., unpublished observations). These findings refer to the first screen; at routine rescreening sensitivity was disappointingly lower at 46% in the first 12 months falling to 35.3% 12–24 months after routine rescreens.

These analyses of sensitivity for cancer detection using interval cancers presenting in screened subjects are inappropriate for estimating the sensitivity for adenoma detection because so few adenomas are diagnosed symptomatically. The number of symptomatic interval adenomas can be counted but probably only represent the tip of the iceberg of all adenomas which are present in the large bowel at that time.

Specificity of Haemoccult

The main reason why Haemoccult has been regarded as a reasonable option for screening is its specificity which is relatively better than that of other faecal occult blood tests. For example in Nottingham [61], 770 (2.1%) of 37 346 screened people had a positive test, among whom exactly half were found to have neoplasia (82 cancers and 303 with adenomas). The remaining 385 were false positives, giving a specificity of 99.0%. The positive predictive value for any neoplasia was 50%, and for cancer was 11%.

Mandel et al. [35] reported a specificity of 97.7% when using unrehydrated Haemoccult but this dropped to 90.4% with rehydrated testing. Specificities as low as this, which involve undertaking colonoscopy in 10% of people without neoplasia, pose a very large burden on asymptomatic people, and use a large volume of health resources. Moreover in a programme involving routine repeat screens, the problem accumulates over time. During Mandel's 13-year follow-up 38% of people were screened annually, and 28% of those screened biennially had at least one colonoscopy.

Other Faecal Occult Blood Tests

A number of newer FOBTs have now been developed, some (e.g. Haemoccult SENSA) being based on the same peroxidase reaction as Haemoccult, others (e.g. Hemoquant) providing a quantitative method by assay of the haemporphyrin component of blood, and others (e.g. Hemeselect) being immunochemical tests specific to human haemoglobin. St John et al. [52] compared the above three tests in patients with known colorectal neoplasia and in 1355 screenees. Hemeselect and Haemoccult SENSA gave higher levels of sensitivity for cancers (97.2% and 93.5% respectively) and adenomas (58.0% and 44.4%, respectively) than the other tests, and in the screened subjects the specificity of Hemeselect (97.8%) was higher than that of Haemoccult SENSA (96.1%).

Thomas et al. [62] compared Hemeselect and Haemoccult in 350 patients referred for investigation of symptoms. Hemeselect had a sensitivity for cancers of 94% compared with Haemoccult's 58%. Similarly its sensitivity for adenomas (66.6%) was also higher than that of Haemoccult 33.3%. Robinson et al. [50] compared these same two tests in screening 4078 subjects aged 50–75 years. Nine cancers were detected, all positive to Hemeselect but only one positive to Haemoccult. Of 49 patients who had adenomas, 48 were positive on Hemeselect but only eight on Haemoccult (there may of course have been many more adenomas undetected by either test). The specificity of Hemeselect was 94.1%, compared with 99.5% for Haemoccult, but the relatively larger yield of cancers from Hemeselect screening meant that its positive predictive value for cancer detection was actually higher than that of Haemoccult (6.2% versus 5.5%). Further investigation of Hemeselect as a screening test may be warranted.

Other Possible Screening Tests for Colorectal Neoplasia

Symptom questionnaires

The symptoms of large bowel cancer include altered bowel habit (either diarrhoea or constipation), rectal bleeding, abdominal pain, abdominal mass, weight loss) and are frequently thought unimportant both by patients and by general practitioners, with consequent delays in diagnosis. It is possible that greater awareness might promote diagnosis at an early stage although Holliday and Hardcastle [24] found no association between duration of symptoms and stage.

Silman et al. [58] investigated screening by symptom questionnaire in 1805 working men and women aged over 50 years. The findings were compared with those of Haemoccult testing in the same individuals. The proportion with one or more symptoms was 12% and all of these and an additional 15 subjects with positive Haemoccult tests were investigated by flexible sigmoidoscopy and barium enema. No cancers were found but seven people had adenomas larger than 10 mm. All of these had at least one symptom, and six were Haemoccult positive. The combination of a positive Haemoccult and at least one symptom gave a positive predictive value for adenoma detection of 46%.

A symptom questionnaire in a rather older population (45–74 years) was not so successful [17]. When compared with the findings of Haemoccult testing in the same individuals, two out of four cancer patients and three out of four patients with adenomas had no symptoms. Thus it seems that symptom questionnaires are likely to be both less sensitive and less specific than FOBT screening.

Ultrasonography

Ultrasonography, with instillation of water into the colon, has been compared with colonoscopy in symptomatic patients, and found to have a sensitivity of 94% for colonic cancers and 80% for adenomas [33]. However, its use in screening is limited by the fact that it cannot visualise the rectum, and in this study, patients required sedation before instillation of 1500 ml of water. At present therefore it cannot be regarded as a suitable test for screening.

Faecal DNA Analysis

A screening method which may prove feasible in the future is a battery of DNA analyses to detect genetic mutations in neoplastic cells in stools [32]. Already it has been shown that K-*ras* oncogene mutations can be detected [57], although because they are not present in all tumours, sensitivity is only 33%. Other potentially detectable genetic alterations include p53 [50] and DCC, but genetic alterations associated with loss of alleles are not detectable by current methods.

Digital Rectal Examination

As seen in Chapter 7, digital rectal examination of asymptomatic men is widely used in screening for prostate cancer. Clearly it also has the potential for detecting low rectal cancers, but at best could have a sensitivity of only around 25%.

The Acceptability of Screening

Given the natural distaste of most people for faeces, one of the most important factors to consider in screening for colorectal neoplasia is the acceptability of the method. Where sigmoidoscopy screening has been available, but where people have not been positively invited, uptake levels are low. For example, in a health maintenance organisation in the United States in which sigmoidoscopy screening was encouraged it was found that over a 10 year period only 24% of people aged over 45 years had had at least one screening sigmoidoscopy and 10% had had more than one [55]. In one small UK study, where a general practitioner invited people aged over 50 years to have flexible sigmoidoscopy, a remarkably high acceptance of 70% was achieved (Verne, personal communication). But other UK studies, inviting people through their general practitioner, have had response rates of less than 30% (K. Vellacott, personal communication). Even in Nordic countries where response to screening is usually higher, only 36% of subjects in Gothenburg, Sweden and 40% of subjects in Odense, Denmark accepted sigmoidoscopy. The need for bowel preparation may deter some people from accepting sigmoidoscopy and comparisons of the acceptability of oral laxative regimes and self-administered enemas are needed.

Faecal occult blood testing may be more acceptable, although again, the incentive of a personal invitation seems to be necessary. In a health maintenance organisation, with a recommendation for screening but no invitation, 43% of people over 50 years had had at least one FOBT within 5 years [56]. In the Danish Haemoccult trial [31], 67% of 30 970 people accepted the first screening invitation, and 2 years later 61% complied with routine screening. In Nottingham, UK [61], 54% of 69 453 individuals accepted the first invitation, and 80% of responders to the first screen accepted routine rescreening. The latter study has investigated factors affecting compliance [18], and has also tried out various types of invitation [48] concluding that a letter from the person's general practitioner achieves the highest response. A randomised controlled trial, also in the UK, compared compliance with a mailed Haemoccult test, an appointment to attend the general practice nurse where a Haemoccult test was then offered, and an offer of a Haemoccult test made by the general practitioner when the person was consulting for some other condition [43]. Compliance was highest (57%) in the latter group, intermediate (49%) in the appointment group and lowest (38%) in the group sent the Haemoccult test by post. The inclusion, or not, of a carefully designed educational booklet with all three invitation methods had no effect on compliance. Hobbs et al. [22] also found that opportunistic screening, when an eligible person consulted for some other complaint, achieved a 56% response. But overall coverage of course depended on the proportion of the target population who consulted; over a 2-year period only 26% of the target population had been screened. This study also noted the customary finding that acceptance of screening fell off with increasing age (although it was also low in the youngest age group, 40–49 years), and was lower in an inner city area than a suburban area.

The Effectiveness of Screening

Sigmoidoscopy Screening

Evidence on the effectiveness of sigmoidoscopy screening is available from four types of study. First there are studies which have followed-up sigmoidoscoped patients who have had adenomas removed and compared their subsequent incidence of cancer with an expected incidence rate.

Murakam et al. [41] followed up 136 people who had had polyps removed and 305 people who had had a polyp diagnosed (either endoscopically or radiographically) but not removed, for a mean period of 6 years. Two cancers subsequently developed in the polypectomy group and nine in the non-polypectomy group. When compared with the expected incidence in the general population derived from the cancer registry, the polypectomy group had a significantly increased relative risk of 2.3 and the non-polypectomy group of 8.0, confirming the increased risk associated with polyps. However, the risk of subsequent cancer in the polypectomy patients relative to the non-polypectomy patients was 0.3 (95% CI 0.1–2.1). Although not statistically significant this certainly suggests a protective effect of polypectomy particularly since the polypectomy patients were more likely to have had large polyps with unfavourable prognostic characteristics.

In another study, which followed-up for 30 years, of 1618 subjects who had had rectal and sigmoid adenomas removed via rigid sigmoidoscopy, 14 (0.9%) subsequently developed rectal cancer [5]. This incidence did not differ significantly from that derived from cancer registry data in the same population, but using Stryker et al.'s [60] estimate of risk it was estimated that at least 80 cancers would have been expected. Moreover 11 of the 14 cancers that developed had had incomplete excision of their adenoma, and the three cases with complete excision of the earlier adenoma arose more than 17 years later. The incidence of cancer proximal to the reach of rigid sigmoidoscopy was significantly greater than that expected in the general population but the increased risk was concentrated entirely in patients who had had a rectal adenoma larger than 1 cm or with a villous histology. On the basis of this study, Atkin et al. [4] suggest that a single sigmoidoscopy at age 55 to 64 could identify and remove a high proportion of potentially premalignant adenomas within reach of the sigmoidoscope, and, by colonoscoping individuals with a large or villous adenoma, also remove a high proportion of those in the proximal colon.

Similarly, Jorgensen et al. [26] in a follow-up of 1056 patients who had had an adenoma removed and who, on colonoscopy started the follow-up period with a "clean" colon, found that over periods of up to 8 years (median 4.3 years), 10 colorectal cancers subsequently developed. This number did not differ significantly from the expected incidence from cancer registry data, nor from the expected conversion rate for all adenomas from Eide's [15] study. However, on the basis of the risk estimates in the latter, the risk of progression of large ($\geq$ 10 mm) and/or severely dysplastic adenomas was reduced by 85 to 90%. The 10 cancers included three in which repeated piecemeal attempts to remove a sessile adenoma were required, and one which was found incidentally in a haemorrhoid. This study differs from that of Atkin et al. [5], in that all the subjects were under regular colonoscopic surveillance, during the course of which 590 further adenomatous polyps were removed in 287 patients. The authors urge caution about their conclusions because of the relatively small size of the study and short period of follow-up.

These adenoma follow-up studies provide evidence in support of the adenoma–carcinoma sequence and of the level of protection which might be achieved in adenoma-bearing patients. However, because they focus only on the latter, not on the whole population, among whom some cancers may develop in people who do not pass through a detectable adenoma phase, they do not measure the degree of protection achieved by population screening.

The second type of evidence addresses this issue by comparing cancer incidence and mortality in a population screened by sigmoidoscopy with the expected incidence and mortality rate in people of the same age and sex distribution in the general (presumed unscreened) population, derived from cancer registration and mortality statistics. In an early screening programme, in which 21 000 volunteers over the age of 45 years were offered annual screening by rigid sigmoidoscopy, it was reported that the subsequent incidence of rectal cancer was only 15% of that expected [19]. However, a later analysis of data from this study disputed the estimate of incidence from which the expected number had originally been derived, and concluded that the cumulative number of cancers in the screened population (including those detected by earlier screens) was similar to the number expected [39].

The third type of study is a randomised controlled trial of screening. There are two studies which are relevant but neither provide a clear answer. The first is a randomised controlled trial of a multiphasic health screening package in a US Health Maintenance Organization (HMO). A total of 10 000 people enrolled in the HMO were randomised to be invited to undergo annual multiphasic screening or to a control group who could request it but were not invited [11]. Rigid sigmoidoscopy was one of the tests included in the package but required the subject to make a separate appointment from that for the main battery of tests. About 60% of the invited group and 20% of the controls underwent multiphasic check-ups but the proportions who had sigmoidoscopy are not reported.

After 11 years a statistically significant reduction in colorectal cancer deaths (five in the intervention group, 18 in the controls) was found [11]. However, the researchers subsequently cast doubt on whether this finding could be attributed to screening [54]. A number of other explanations are possible, including a higher incidence of colorectal cancer in the control group both before entry to the trial and subsequently; the fact that there was only a difference of four cases in the numbers diagnosed by screening in the two groups (seven in the intervention group, three in the controls); and the possibility that in a trial such as this, which investigated differences in death rates for 34 separate conditions, one or two comparisons might be expected to be significant by chance.

The second randomised controlled trial was a study of faecal occult blood testing [35], which is described in greater detail below. It is of relevance to the effectiveness of endoscopy because 38% of the group who were offered annual FOBT and 28% of the group offered biennial FOBT had at least one colonoscopy during the 13 years of the trial. It is likely that several non-bleeding polyps were identified and removed during these colonoscopies and that this may have resulted in a decreased incidence of cancer attributable to the colonoscopy rather than the FOBT, although there was no significant difference in incidence between the three groups. During the last 5 years of the trial the cumulative incidence of cancer increased less in the screened groups than the control group. Interpretation of the extent to which colonoscopy contributed to polyp removal, and thence to reduced incidence, requires more detail than is yet published on the timing of colonoscopy, the number of polypectomies, and the number of years of follow-up.

The fourth type of study addressing the effectiveness of sigmoidoscopy is the case-control method. Two such studies have been reported, both aimed at showing whether screening sigmoidoscopy protects against death from colorectal cancer (reduced mortality) rather than against development of colorectal cancer (reduced incidence). Thus the mechanism for protection in these studies could be the identification of curable cancers, or the identification of premalignant adenomas, or both. Selby et al. [55] conducted a study in the same HMO which had had the multiphasic health screening programme already mentioned. They took as cases 261 people who had died of rectal and distal colon cancers between 1971 and 1988, and 868 controls matched for age and sex. The history of sigmoidoscopy screening in cases and controls up to the date of diagnosis of the case was then compared. Only 9% of the cases had undergone screening compared with 24% of the controls. After adjusting for potential confounding variables their conclusion was that the risk of death from a cancer within reach of the sigmoidoscope was reduced by 59% in screened subjects relative to unscreened.

As discussed in Chapter 1, case-control studies normally suffer from a selection bias in that subjects with the greatest risk of death are also those least likely to avail themselves of screening. However, in this study it was found that the risk of death from colon cancer proximal to the reach of sigmoidoscopy was no different in screened or unscreened people, arguing against any selection bias in this study. The level of protection was calculated separately according to the number of years between the most recent screening examination, and the diagnosis of the fatal cancer. It was found to be as high 9–10 years before diagnosis, as within 1–4 years of diagnosis. This suggests that sigmoidoscopy screening can protect both by removal of adenomas and by removal of early cancers, and supports the hypothesis that a single sigmoidoscopy can give long-term protection [4].

The second case-control study [42] was also conducted in a health maintenance organisation, and included 66 cases who had died of colorectal cancer and 196 matched controls. Screening histories included sigmoidoscopy, FOBTs and rectal examination. The odds ratio (OR) of a person screened by sigmoidoscopy dying, relative to that of an unscreened person, was 0.21 (95% CI 0.08–0.52). When divided by subsite the OR for rectal and distal colon cancer was 0.05 (95% CI 0.01–0.43), but for proximal colon cancer it was also reduced, although not significantly so (OR 0.36, 95% CI 0.11–1.20). These odds ratios were adjusted for FOBTs and digital rectal examinations, which, when similarly adjusted for sigmoidoscopy screens, had no effect on the risk of death. No information on duration of protection was reported.

Faecal Occult Blood Screening

Because of its cheapness, simplicity and presumed greater acceptability, FOBT screening has been used to a greater extent than sigmoidoscopy in studies of the effectiveness of screening based on representative populations rather than on volunteers. But in view of the poor sensitivity of FOBTs for detecting adenomas, these studies have so far focused mainly on the identification and removal of cancers, and therefore on reduction of colorectal cancer mortality as their end-point.

Selby et al. [56], in their Health Maintenance Organization in which FOBT screening had been encouraged, matched 496 patients who had died from a colorectal cancer with 727 controls, and compared their histories of FOBT screening, adjusting for the number of rectal examinations, sigmoidoscopies and other confounders. Their results indicate an approximate 25% reduction in risk of death from colorectal cancer in subjects screened every 1–2 years but this was not statistically significant.

In Germany, annual Haemoccult testing is available for people over 45 years as part of a free government health insurance scheme. Wahrendorf et al. [65] conducted a similar case-control study in the state of Saarland identifying 522 people aged 45–74 years who had died from colorectal cancer. Because of restrictive legislation on the confidentiality of medical records, the researchers had to find suitable controls from each case's general practitioner, and, for women, also from her gynaecologist because most FOBT screening is done in association with cervical smears. A total of 372 cases were matched with five controls each, and the number of screening FOBTs within 3 years prior to diagnosis of the case recorded for each. For men, no protective effect was found but the participation of men in the screening programme is low, estimated at no more than 13% during the period under study. For women on the other hand, whose participation was higher (up to 23%), a statistically significant 57% reduction in risk of colorectal cancer death in screened subjects compared to unscreened was found (OR 0.43, 95% CI 0.27–0.68). It was not possible in this study to adjust for possible confounding variables and, therefore, some of the difference may be attributable to selection bias.

A number of large population-based randomised controlled trials of faecal occult blood screening are in progress. In Nottingham, 178 000 people aged 50–74 years have been randomised to a group offered 2-yearly faecal occult blood tests or to a control group [61]. In Denmark, Kronborg et al. [29] have similarly randomised 62 000 people, and Kewenter et al. [28], in Sweden, have randomised 51 000 people aged 60–64 years [28]. In Minnesota [9], 46550 volunteers aged 50–80 years have been randomised to a group offered screening annually, a group offered it biennially and a control group. All of these studies are designed to compare mortality from colorectal cancer in the intervention group with that in the control group.

The Minnesota study reported its mortality findings 13 years from the start of the trial [35]. The cumulative mortality from colorectal cancer was 5.88 deaths per 1000 persons in the annually screened group, significantly lower than the rate of 8.83 deaths per 1000 in the control group. However, the colorectal cancer mortality rate in the biennially screened group was 8.33 per 1000, only marginally lower than the controls. Half of the 354 cancers in the annually screened group were detected at screening, the remainder presenting as interval cancers at varying intervals after the last negative screen. Only 39% of the 368 cancers in the biennially screened group were screen-detected; the distribution of interval cancers arising in successive years after a negative screen is not reported so it is not possible to compare the sensitivity of a 1-year interval with that of a 2-year interval. But 60% of the biennially screened group completed all scheduled screenings compared with only 46% of the annually screened group. When examined by stage the principal difference between the groups was a 50% reduction in Stage D tumours in the annually screened group compared with controls. The biennially screened group had 39% fewer Stage D tumours but 20% more Stage C tumours, compared with the control group.

The conclusion of this study is that annual faecal occult blood screening can reduce mortality by 33%, but since rehydrated Haemoccult tests were used specificity was low, and nearly two-fifths of the annually screened group had at least one colonoscopy. How much of the reduced mortality is due to colonoscopy is unknown, and the lack of an intermediate effect in the biennially screened group is unexplained.

Preliminary mortality results from the Danish study have been published and show a non-significant 27% reduction in the intervention group compared with controls (37 deaths compared with 51) [29]. This is remarkable since the incidence of Stage D tumours in the intervention group was 13% higher than in the controls. The other European trials have not yet published mortality data, but in preliminary reports [28, 61], both have found a higher incidence of Stage A tumours in the intervention group, but also a slightly higher incidence of Stage D. The follow-up time in these studies is relatively short and one would not expect a reduction in advanced cancers to appear for some years after the introduction of the screening programme, so further years of observation are required.

Disadvantages and Costs

As with screening for other cancer sites it is possible that awareness of screening, implying concern about vulnerability to colorectal cancer, may of itself cause anxiety, but there has been little research in this area. Mant [37] found that around 20% of people screened by FOBT were distressed by the screening invitation but 98% felt it had been worthwhile. The anxiety induced by a positive screening result, particularly one which eventually turns out to be a false positive, must be counted as one of the unwanted side-effects of screening. In Mant et al.'s [37] study, 37 out of

54 (69%) subjects with false positive results were worried that they might have cancer, 12 (22%) being very concerned. Weller et al. [67] reported similar findings following FOBT and noted that 31% remained worried even after a negative diagnostic work-up.

Faecal occult blood testing entails no risk of physical morbidity but the same is not true of sigmoidoscopy screening. Maule [38] noted that 45% of flexible sigmoid-oscopies were terminated before reaching 60 cm because of discomfort or pain, and that this was commoner in women (55%) than in men (32%).

Complications from endoscopic polypectomy including bleeding and perforation have been reported from patients undergoing colonoscopy, who are under sedation, but these side-effects are less severe and less frequent for removal of polyps under 2 cm [26], and presumably are also less likely in unsedated patients undergoing flexible sigmoidoscopy. Jorgensen et al. [26] noted that perforation of the sigmoid colon had occurred in eight patients in their adenoma surveillance programme out of 3959 diagnostic colonoscopies; one patient died from a myocardial infarct 5 days after surgical repair of the perforation. Polypectomy also entails some iatrogenic risk; out of 1801 polypectomies in the same series, there were three perforations (one of whom died) and one haemorrhage necessitating surgery to transfix the bleeding site. In addition, there were 24 minor complications not requiring surgery. Thus in this large series, the procedure-related mortality was 0.3 per 1000, the serious complication rate 2 per 1000 and the minor complication rate 4 per 1000. In balancing non-fatal complications against the presumed benefits of screening, their occurrence needs to be documented – both those arising as a result of screening, and those which would have arisen anyway, during investigation of symptoms.

Resource costs have been measured mainly in relation to FOBT screening [66, 67]. In the UK in 1989, considering only the first screening round, the cost per person screened was £5.00 and per cancer detected £2700 [66]. Sensitivity analyses showed that performance variables such as compliance and detection rates have a much greater influence on total cost than do variations in the costs of resources. In Australia, where colonoscopy is relatively more expensive, the proportion that tests positive is the most important variable [67].

Ultimately, of course, it is the extra cost per cancer or per death avoided, or per quality adjusted life-year gained that should inform judgements about whether screening programmes give good value for money, but these must await the findings of randomised controlled trials. Atkin et al. [4] estimate that their sigmoidoscopy screening programme would cost £5500 per cancer prevented or £8500 per death avoided and that savings of treatment costs could go a long way to offset these costs. Use of trained non-medical staff to undertake screening would also defray costs [38]. A more sophisticated model [63] estimates that annual screening by FOBT starting at age 65 years would cost $US 35 000 per year of life gained.

Conclusions

There is accumulating evidence that the natural history of colorectal cancer is amenable to intervention by identification of premalignant adenomas and early cancers. But, unlike the situation with development of breast cancer screening, clear unequivocal evidence of the extent of reduction in incidence and mortality which can be achieved is still lacking. This still awaits the outcome of population-based randomised controlled trials. Several are in progress using faecal occult blood screening, and two, using sigmoidoscopy screening, are planned [4, 47].

Faecal occult blood testing is more acceptable to the general public than sigmoidoscopy, but lacks sensitivity for cancer detection unless it is rehydrated which leads to unacceptable loss of specificity. Sigmoidoscopy, however, has much greater sensitivity and has the additional advantage of enabling detection and removal of adenomas; this means that perhaps just a single examination at around age 60 years might give considerable protection against future cancer, and if this were proven to be true would probably increase acceptability.

Despite the optimism that it may be beneficial, it is premature to advocate widespread screening of the general population until its benefits and costs are more clearly established.

References

1. Adami H-O (1988) Aspects of descriptive epidemiology and survival in colorectal cancer. Scand J Gastroenterol. Suppl 149:6–20.
2. Ahlquist DA, McGill DB, Schwartz S, Taylor WF, Owen RA (1985) Fecal blood levels in health and disease. A study using Hemoquant. Gastroenterology 82:891–898.
3. Armstrong B, Doll R (1975) Environmental factors and cancer incidence in different countries, with special reference to dietary practices. Int J Cancer 15:617–631.
4. Atkin WS, Cuzick J, Northover JMA, Whynes DK (1993) Prevention of colorectal cancer by once-only sigmoidoscopy. Lancet 341:736–740.
5. Atkin WS, Morson BC, Cuzick J (1992) Long-term risk of colorectal cancer after excision of rectosigmoid adenomas. N Engl J Med 326:658–662.
6. Bingham SA (1990) Diet and large bowel cancer. J R Soc Med 83:420–422.
7. Black RJ, Sharp L, Kendrick SW (1993) Trends in cancer survival in Scotland, 1968–1990. Information and Statistics Division, ISD Publications, Edinburgh.
8. Burkitt DP (1969) Related disease – related cause. Lancet ii:1229–1231.
9. Church TR, Mandel JS, Bond JH et al. (1991) Colon cancer control study: status and current issues. In: Miller AB, Chamberlain J, Day NE, Hakama M, Prorok PC (eds) Cancer screening. UICC project on evaluation of screening for cancer. Cambridge University Press, Cambridge, pp 83–105.
10. Clark JC, Collan Y, Eide TJ et al. (1985) Prevalence of polyps in an autopsy series from areas with varying incidence of large-bowel cancer. Int J Cancer 36:179–186.
11. Dales LG, Friedman GD, Collen MF (1979) Evaluating periodic multiphasic health checkups: a controlled study. J Chron Dis 32:385–404.
12. Doran J, Hardcastle JD (1982) Bleeding patterns in colorectal cancer: the effect of aspirin and the implications for faecal occult blood testing. Br J Surg 69:711–713.
13. Donohue JH, Nelson H (1992) The current status of adjuvant therapy for colon cancer. Adv Surg 25:223–257.
14. Eide TJ (1983) Remnants of adenomas in colorectal carcinomas. Cancer 51:1866–1872.
15. Eide TJ (1986) Risk of colorectal cancer in adenoma-bearing individuals within a

defined population. Int J Cancer 38:173–176.

16. Farrands PA, Hardcastle JD (1983) Accuracy of occult blood tests over a six-day period. Clin Oncol 9:217–225.

17. Farrands PA, Hardcastle JD (1984) Colorectal screening by a self-completion questionnaire. Gut 25:445–447.

18. Farrands PA, Hardcastle JD, Chamberlain J (1984) Factors affecting compliance with screening for colorectal cancer. Community Med 6:12–19.

19. Gilbertsen VA, Nelms JM (1978) The prevention of invasive cancer of the rectum. Cancer 41: 1137–1139.

20. Hardcastle JD, Chamberlain J, Sheffield J et al. (1989) Randomised controlled trial of faecal occult blood screening for colorectal cancer. Results of the first 107 349 subjects. Lancet i:1160–1164.

21. Hill MJ (1989) Experimental studies of fat, fibre and calories in carcinogenesis. In: Miller AB, Veronesi U (eds) Diet and the aetiology of cancer. European School of Oncology Monograph. Springer-Verlag, Berlin, pp 31–38.

22. Hobbs FDR, Cherry RC, Fielding JWL, Pike L, Holder R (1992) Acceptability of opportunistic screening for occult gastrointestinal blood loss. Br Med J 304:483–486.

23. Hoff G, Foerster A, Vatn MH et al. (1986) Epidemiology of polyps in the rectum and colon. Recovery and evaluation of unresected polyps 2 years after detection. Scand J Gastroenterol 21:853–862.

24. Holliday HW, Hardcastle JD (1979) Delay in diagnosis and treatment of symptomatic colorectal cancer. Lancet i:309–311.

25. Jahn H, Jorgensen OD, Kronborg O et al. (1992) Can Haemoccult II replace colonoscopy in surveillance after radical surgery for colorectal cancer and after polypectomy? Dis Colon Rectum 35:253–256.

26. Jorgensen OD, Kronborg O, Fenger C (1993) The Funen adenoma follow-up study. Incidence and death from colorectal carcinoma in an adenoma surveillance program. Scand J Gastroenterol 28:869–874.

27. Kee F, Wilson RH, Gilliland R et al. (1992) Changing site distribution of colorectal cancer. Br Med J 305:158.

28. Kewenter J, Bjork S, Haglind E, Smith L, Svanvik J, Ahren C (1988) Screening and rescreening for colorectal cancer. A controlled trial of fecal occult blood testing in 27 700 subjects. Cancer 62:645–651.

29. Kronborg O, Fenger C, Olsen J, Bech K, Sondergaard O (1989) Repeated screening for colorectal cancer with fecal occult blood test. Scand J Gastroenterol 24:599–606.

30. Kronborg O, Fenger C, Sondergaard O, Pedersen KM, Olsen J (1987) Initial mass screening for colorectal cancer with fecal occult blood test. A prospective randomised study at Funen in Denmark. Scand J Gastroenterol 22:677–686.

31. Kronborg O, Fenger C, Olsen J (1991) Interim report on a randomised trial of screening for colorectal cancer with Hemoccult-II. In: Miller AB, Chamberlain J, Day NE, Hakama M, Prorok PC (eds) Cancer screening. UICC project on evaluation of screening for cancer. Cambridge University Press, Cambridge, pp 126–130.

32. Lancet (1992) Screening for colorectal cancer by stool DNA analysis (Editorial). Lancet 339:1141–1142.

33. Limberg B (1990) Diagnosis of large bowel tumours by colonic sonography. Lancet 335:144–146.

34. Macrae FA, St. John DJ (1982) Relationship between patterns of bleeding and Haemoccult sensitivity in patients with colorectal cancers or adenomas. Gastroenterology 82:891.

35. Mandel JS, Bond JH, Church TR et al. (1993) Reducing mortality from colorectal cancer by screening for fecal occult blood. N Engl J Med 328:1365–1371.
36. Manning AM, Williams AC, Game SM, Paraskeva C (1991) Differential sensitivity of human colonic adenoma and carcinoma cells to transforming growth factor β (TGF-β): conversion of an adenoma cell line to a tumorigenic phenotype is accompanied by a reduced response to the inhibitory effects of TGF-β. Oncogene 6:1471–1476.
37. Mant D, Fitzpatrick R, Hogg A et al. (1990) Experiences of patients with false positive results from colorectal cancer screening. Br J Gen Pract 40:423–425.
38. Maule WF (1994) Screening for colorectal cancer by nurse endoscopists. N Engl J Med 330:183–187.
39. Miller AB (1988) Review of sigmoidoscopic screening for colorectal cancer. In: Chamberlain J, Miller AB (eds) Screening for gastrointestinal cancer. International Union Against Cancer, Hans Huber, Toronto, pp 3–8.
40. Morson BC (1976) Genesis of colorectal cancer. Clin Gastroenterol 5:505–524.
41. Murakam R, Tsukama H, Kanamori S et al. (1990) Natural history of colorectal polyps and the effect of polypectomy on occurrence of subsequent cancer. Int J Cancer 46:159–164.
42. Newcomb PA, Norfleet RG, Storer BE, Surawicz TS, Marcus PM (1992) Screening sigmoidoscopy and colorectal cancer mortality. J Natl Cancer Inst 84:1572–1575.
43. Nichols S, Koch E, Lallemand RC et al. (1986) Randomised trial of compliance with screening for colorectal cancer. Br Med J 293:107–110.
44. Office of Population Censuses and Surveys (1993) Mortality statistics, 1992. Series DH2, No. 19. HMSO, London.
45. Office of Population Censuses and Surveys (1993) Cancer statistics. Registrations of cancer diagnosed in 1987, England and Wales. Series MBI, No. 20. HMSO, London.
46. Osmond C, Gardner M, Acheson ED, Adelstein AM (1983) Trends in cancer mortality 1951–1980. Office of Population Censuses and Surveys, Series DH, No. 11. HMSO, London.
47. Prorok PC, Byar DP, Smart CR, Baker SG, Connor RJ (1991) Evaluation of screening for prostate, lung, and colorectal cancers. In: Miller AB, Chamberlain J, Day NE, Hakama M, Prorok PC (eds) Cancer screening. UICC project on evaluation of screening for cancer. Cambridge University Press, Cambridge, pp 300–320.
48. Pye G, Christie M, Chamberlain J, Moss SM, Hardcastle JD (1988) A comparison of methods for increasing compliance within a general practitioner-based screening project for colorectal cancer and the effect on practitioner workload. J Epidemiol Community Health 42(1):66-71.
49. Robinson MHE, Thomas WM, Hardcastle JD, Chamberlain J, Mangham CM (1993) Change towards earlier stage at presentation of colorectal cancer. Br J Surg 80:1610–1612.
50. Robinson MHE, Marks CG, Farrands PA, Thomas WM, Hardcastle JD (1994) Population screening for colorectal cancer: comparison between a guaiac and immunological faecal occult blood test. Br J Surg 81:448–451.
51. Robinson MHE, Kronborg O, Williams CB et al. (1995) Faecal occult blood testing and colonoscopy in the surveillance of subjects at high risk of colorectal neoplasia. Br J Surg 82:318–320.
52. St John DJB, Young GP, Alexeyeff MA, Deacon MC et al. (1993) Evaluation of new occult blood tests for detection of colorectal neoplasia. Gastroenterology 104:1661–1668.
53. Sauar J, Hoff G, Hausken T et al. (1992) Colonoscopic screening examination of

relatives of patients with colorectal cancer II, relations between tumour characteristics and the presence of polyps. Scand J Gastroenterol 27:667–672.

54. Selby JV, Friedman GD, Collen MF (1988) Sigmoidoscopy and mortality from colorectal cancer: the Kaiser Permanente multiphasic evaluation study. J Clin Epidemiol 41(5):427–434.

55. Selby JV, Friedman GD, Quesenberry CP Jr, Weiss NS (1992) A case-control study of screening sigmoidoscopy and mortality from colorectal cancer. N Engl J Med 326:653–657.

56. Selby JV, Friedman GD, Quesenberry CP Jr, Weiss NS (1993) Effect of fecal occult blood testing on mortality from colorectal cancer. A case-control study. Ann Intern Med 118:1–6.

57. Sidransky D, Tokino T, Hamilton S et al. (1992) Identification of ras oncogene mutations in the stool of patients with curable colorectal tumours. Science 256:102–105.

58. Silman AJ, Mitchell P, Nicholls RJ et al. (1983) Self-reported dark red bleeding as a marker comparable with occult blood testing in screening for large bowel neoplasms. Br J Surg 70:721–724.

59. Stower MJ, Hardcastle JD (1985) Five year survival of 1115 patients with colorectal cancer. Eur J Surg Oncol 11:119–123.

60. Stryker SJ, Wolff BG, Culp CE, Libbe SD, Ilstrup DM, MacCarty RL (1987) Natural history of untreated colonic polyps. Gastroenterology 93:1009–1013.

61. Thomas WM, Hardcastle JD (1991) An update on the Nottingham trial of faecal occult blood screening for colorectal carcinoma. In: Miller AB, Chamberlain J, Day NE, Hakama M, Prorok PC (eds) Cancer screening. UICC project on evaluation of screening for cancer. Cambridge University Press, Cambridge, pp 106–115.

62. Thomas WM, Hardcastle JD, Jackson J, Pye G (1992) Chemical and immunological testing for faecal occult blood: a comparison of two tests in symptomatic patients. Br J Cancer 65:618–620.

63. US Congress, Office of Technology Assessment (1990) Costs and effectiveness of colorectal cancer screening in the elderly – background paper, OTA-BP-H-74. US Government Printing Office, Washington, D.C.

64. Vogelstein B, Fearon ER, Hamilton SR et al. (1988) Genetic alterations during colorectal tumour development. N Engl J Med 319:525–532.

65. Wahrendorf J, Robra B-P, Wiebelt H, Oberhausen R, Willand M, Dhom G (1993) Effectiveness of colorectal cancer screening: results from a population-based case-control evaluation in Saarland, Germany. Eur J Cancer Prev 2:221–227.

66. Walker A, Whynes DK, Chamberlain JO, Hardcastle JD (1991) The cost of screening for colorectal cancer. J Epidemiol and Community Health 45:220–224.

67. Weller D, Moss J, Hiller J, Edwards J, Thomas D (1994) Screening for colorectal cancer – what are the costs? Int J Tech Ass Health Care.

68. Williams AR, Balasooriya BD, Day DW (1982) Polyps and cancer in the large bowel: a necropsy study in Liverpool. Gut 23:835–842.

5 – Early Detection of Malignant Melanoma of the Skin

Jane Melia

Introduction

Both the mortality and incidence of malignant melanoma of the skin are low in most countries compared with other cancers. The importance of the disease lies in the fact that it affects all adult age groups and both incidence and mortality have increased markedly during recent decades in caucasian populations.

In England and Wales a total of 1142 deaths from melanoma occurred in 1992. The mortality rate was 1.6 per 100000 in males and 1.3 per 100000 in females adjusted to the world standard population [56]. Death from melanoma was rare before the age of 25 but thereafter increased with age in both sexes to over 9.0 per 100000 in males and 7.5 per 100000 in females aged 75 or more. The rates in England and Wales are similar to those in several European and Scandinavian countries. A comprehensive comparison of international trends in mortality [14] shows that the highest rates were found in Australia and New Zealand where the 1985 world-standardised rates in 30–74 year olds averaged 8.3 per 100000 in men and 5.4 per 100000 in women. During the past two decades the mortality rate has increased in many countries by 50% to 100%.

The incidence rates of malignant melanoma tend to be higher in women than men, in contrast to the mortality rates. In England and Wales in 1987 there were 1133 new registered cases in men and 2006 cases in women yielding world standardised rates of 3.5 and 5.6 per 100000, respectively [55]. The relation to age is similar to that for mortality with the disease being rare before age 25 and increasing in older age groups. There is wide variation in incidence rates between countries [14], the rates being highest in Australasia with world standardised rates in 30–74 year olds in 1985 of 47 per 100000 in men and 42 per 100000 in women in New South Wales, Australia. Incidence rates have risen more steeply than mortality rates but part of this increase is likely to be due to improving ascertainment of cases by cancer registries.

Evidence from epidemiological studies has indicated that exposure to ultraviolet radiation from the sun is involved in the aetiology of the disease and that the fashion for sunbathing, tanning and holidays abroad has contributed to the rising disease rates. Although there has been concern about depletion of the ozone layer leading to increased exposure to the sun's rays, it is now estimated that this will only result in a small increase in rates compared with that seen in the past few decades [21].

As metastatic melanoma has a poor prognosis and treatment is mainly palliative, the main options for controlling the disease are primary prevention and early detection. Primary prevention aims to alter people's attitude towards sun exposure so that in the long-term both the incidence and mortality from melanoma will be reduced. However, assuming a long latent interval between exposure and development of neoplasia even if primary prevention is effective, it is likely to take 20 or more years before incidence rates will start to change. Early detection aims to diagnose melanoma at an early stage when treatment by simple excision is thought to be effective and thus curb the rising mortality rates. If effective the benefits to mortality could be seen within seven years and early detection has the added attraction that it could benefit a large proportion of the adult population who already carry an increased risk of developing melanoma because of excessive exposure to the sun earlier in their lives, for whom it is already too late for primary prevention to have much effect.

There is evidence from several studies that early stage disease is associated with good prognosis. Breslow [8] showed a strong association between tumour thickness and survival. A summary of data from several studies [47] showed five-year survival rates of 96%–99% for patients with primary melanomas less than 0.76 mm thick, 87–94% for patients with tumours 0.76–1.5 mm thick, 66%–77% for patients with tumours 1.51 – 4.0 mm thick and less than 50% for patients with tumours thicker than 4.0 mm. Some variation in survival may be caused by differences in the type of melanomas and other factors such as body site and sex. In particular estimates of survival of early stage tumours may vary because they include a proportion of non-progressive tumours which would not lead to metastatic disease and a proportion of borderline benign cases.

Natural History

Melanoma is a cancer derived from melanocytes which are usually found in the basal layer of the epidermis. A proportion of melanomas evolve in precursor lesions which include a variety of naevi and lentigo maligna or Hutchinson's melanotic freckle. The exact proportion is unknown because most estimates are based on subjective recall by patients with melanoma. There is a considerable debate about the type of naevi involved and research is needed to assess ways of identifying which type of naevi are most likely to progress to melanoma and would benefit from early excision. Patients with large congenital naevi and similar naevi which appear shortly after birth have an increased incidence of malignant melanoma but the type which could lead to melanoma is uncertain thus making patient management difficult [4]. Many atypical naevi develop during childhood and it has been suggested that the number of naevi increases with increased exposure to UV radiation during this period. Certainly having a large number of naevi in adulthood is one of the main risk factors associated with melanoma although the estimate of risk varies because of the different criteria used to count naevi in the different studies [31, 66]. UV radiation may act as both an initiator and promotor of melanoma in this pathway. The exact mechanism is uncertain but it may include DNA and immunological changes.

Dysplastic naevi have been found in families with a high risk of developing melanoma but there is lack of agreement about the clinical and histological definitions of diagnosis of these naevi. Several families with multiple atypical precursor naevi have shown a high risk of developing melanoma and it is estimated that 6%–10% of all cutaneous melanomas occur in persons with a positive family history of the disease. Genetic studies have shown that melanoma is linked in some families to a dominant gene on chromosome 9p [11] but gene mapping is in its early stages and there may well be other genes, perhaps of low penetrance, involved in the aetiology of the disease.

The period between initiation and development of cancer, and the time that it takes for a non-invasive melanoma to grow into an invasive, potentially metastatic phase is not known. As it is unethical to observe melanomas growing in situ the only other information comes from retrospective studies in which patients were asked when they first noticed their lesion before seeking medical attention. Temoshok et al. [67] found a significant positive correlation between delay in diagnosis and tumour thickness, the longest mean delay being 6 months. In contrast Cassileth et al. [12] found no such correlation but this may have occurred because of different case-mix in the two studies. In one area of the UK 48% of melanoma patients reported that their lesion had been present for one year [70] or more, but the results were not presented by stage. As with other cancers the growth rate will depend on many factors including tumour type, body site, sex of the patient and several other host and external factors.

There are four main types of melanoma. Superficial spreading and nodular melanomas occur in all adult age groups and are thought to be associated with intermittent excessive exposure to the sun. Lentigo malignant melanomas are found mostly in the elderly and are associated with long-term sun exposure. Acral melanomas are found on palms and soles of both white and non-white populations, and as these sites rarely experience excessive sun exposure other aetiological factors such as trauma and viruses have been suggested. Superficial spreading and lentigo malignant melanomas nearly always have a radial growth phase [13] and these are thought to have the potential to grow slowly and thus be amenable to cure by early detection. It is suggested that these types are less likely to arise in existing naevi but first appear as a dark patch or freckle. In contrast nodular and acral melanomas which are more likely to have a vertical growth phase [13] are usually detected when already invasive and thus may be more difficult to prevent by early detection. Survival rates have been found to be better for superficial spreading and lentigo malignant melanoma than for nodular melanoma [44].

The Screening Test for Malignant Melanoma

The detection of melanoma in its early stages relies on certain clinical signs, although these are subject to a certain amount of error even among trained dermatologists. In the UK, a seven point checklist derived from clinical data on patients attending clinics in Glasgow (Table 5.1) [40] was used in the 1980s in two

Table 5.1 Glasgow seven-point check-list [41]

1.	Presence of itch or altered sensation
2.	Diameter of 1 cm or greater
3.	Increasing size
4.	Presence of an irregular or geographical lateral border
5.	Variation in density of black and brown pigment within the lesion
6.	Inflammation
7.	Bleeding or crusting

large-scale health education programmes of the general public [20, 43]. The Glasgow checklist gave equal importance to increasing size, variegation in colour, inflammation, irregular outline, diameter > 1 cm, itch and bleeding. The presence of three or more features was considered suspicious and such cases were recommended for referral to a dermatologist. Subsequent evaluation of the checklist showed that features such as itch were non-specific to melanoma and that requiring a diameter > 1 cm could lead to small early stage melanomas being missed. The checklist underwent two revisions [18, 41]. du Vivier et al. [18] in a study of 100 melanomas reported a low prevalence of the clinical signs of itch, inflammation and diameter > 1 cm from the 1985 checklist and reported that the checklist was particularly poor at identification of nodular melanoma. The latest version (Table 5.2) places emphasis on changes in the lesion, and gives less priority to sensory change. The diameter is reduced to > 7 mm.

Table 5.2 Revised seven-point check-list [41]

Major features

1.	Change in size of previous lesion or obvious growth of new lesion
2.	Irregular shape – asymmetry and an irregular outline of a newly developed pigmented lesion or appearance of this feature in an old lesion
3.	Irregular colour – a variety of shades of brown and black in a new or old lesion

Minor features

4.	Largest diameter 7 mm or greater
5.	Inflammation
6.	Oozing, crusting or bleeding
7.	Change in sensation

In the USA, the ABCD system [39] advises that one of three features of asymmetry, border irregularity, colour irregularity or diameter > 6 mm should be present. The authors found these to be a better predictor of melanoma than the Glasgow checklist recommended by MacKie [40]. In the revised British checklist the diameter of 7 mm recommended by MacKie [41] may need to be adjusted if there is a further shift towards an increase of smaller thin lesions being detected. In Australia, where early detection has been encouraged for many years, one-third of melanomas were found to have diameters 6 mm or less [63]. With emphasis placed on change, some tumours may still be missed as it may be easier to notice an irregularity in border or colour but less easy to be aware of change in a slow growing tumour or one in a less readily observed site on the body, such as the back.

Further work is required to evaluate the revised checklist. The frequency of these signs needs to be studied in the general population, not just in the dermatology clinic which will see mostly lesions selected for referral because of suspicious signs. Moreover studies of the accuracy of clinical diagnosis in referred patients have not necessarily used the check-lists, and their findings with regard to sensitivity, specificity and predictive value are not relevant to screening asymptomatic members of the general public.

Options for Screening

The main options for screening which have been investigated are health education to promote self-screening by the general population and certain types of organised professional screening. Each option is discussed separately because they have very different implications in terms of organisation, uptake, accuracy of the screening test, evaluation and thus overall effectiveness.

Health Education to Promote Self-Screening

Self-screening by the general population has been considered by many to be the most practical and least expensive method of screening compared with professional screening. As the incidence of the disease is low a large proportion of the population would have to be screened to detect just a few melanomas. Self-screening has mostly been promoted through specific health education programmes which have taken place in several countries in Europe, Australasia and the USA.

To develop effective health education which ultimately would help to prevent death from melanoma, various stages in the health education process should be studied. It is important to understand who detects melanoma in the community, why delays occur in seeking medical attention, methods for disseminating the health education message, and accuracy of the clinical signs recommended for use by the general public. It is also important in the planning stage to establish methods for evaluating both short-term and long-term effects of the health education programme.

Who Detects Melanoma?

In the UK a pigmented lesion clinic was started in Southampton in 1981 [64] to reduce delays in referral of patients by GPs to hospital. The mean thickness of the tumour was not significantly lower than among patients referred elsewhere or seen in Southampton in the previous five years. Following on from this research greater emphasis was placed in the UK on educating the general public about the early signs of melanoma to reduce delay between development of a suspect lesion and seeking medical advice. In a study of 202 melanoma cases identified in Tayside, Scotland from 1982 to 1987 several causes of delay in treatment were identified [19]. Patient delay of more than 3 months in seeking medical advice was found for 60% of cases, delay after presentation to the GP was identified for 21% and in 12% an opportunity for earlier diagnosis by the GP had been missed.

The distribution of melanomas by body site probably has an important effect on detection. The most frequent sites are: for women the lower limb and head/face, and for men the trunk and head/neck. In the USA Rigel et al. [60] reported that only one in 14 lesions would be found by partial examination of parts of the body not normally covered by clothing.

In a study in London [18] nearly half of patients presenting with melanoma at a pigmented lesion clinic had come at the insistence of their relatives or friends or because of the family doctor's incidental diagnosis. This is similar to a study in the USA [36]. About 53% of melanomas were self-discovered, 26% by medical providers and the remainder by others. Nearly one-third of cases said that they could not see their own lesion easily and women (66%) were more likely to discover their own lesions than men (42%).

Public Awareness About Melanoma and Clinical Signs

Awareness about melanoma has been studied in Britain and Australia. In Britain, a national survey of melanoma awareness [49] showed over 45% of people knew that melanoma was a skin cancer but those least aware were men, the elderly, those under 20 years, poor socioeconomic groups and those living on their own.

In Australia recognition of the term melanoma was much higher (91%) but many people had misconceptions about the key characteristics [7]. More importantly in a study in New South Wales [28] it was reported that only 32% of people who had observed clinical signs of melanoma had sought medical advice within a recommended period. Among those not seeking advice or delaying, not knowing the importance of early detection of melanoma was found in 30% and not knowing that the sign was serious was found in 49%. As death from melanoma occurs most frequently in men and the elderly, in the future any health education campaigns should target these specific subsets of the population to improve knowledge about the early clinical signs.

The public's recognition of clinical signs using the Glasgow checklist and revised version has been assessed in three studies. Keefe et al. [33] reported that patients had a lower predictive value than the dermatologists for recognising melanoma. The authors concluded that improving the public's recognition of an irregular margin would aid the early detection of melanoma. Higgins et al. [30] in a study of benign lesions found the revised checklist [18] to be less specific than the 1985 version, and that, even among lesions considered to be suspicious by patients using the original checklist, 94% of cases were reported benign by dermatologists.

Organisation of Health Education Programmes

In the UK two large-scale health education programmes have been launched to promote the early detection of melanoma by the general public. The aim in both programmes was to reduce patient delay in seeking medical advice because patient delay was one of the main factors which had been associated with late stage presentation [64]. Although the health education advised people about the early signs of melanoma these were different from self-screening programmes because they did not teach regular whole-body examinations for suspicious lesions or advise about the frequency of screening. The campaigns, which took place in the West of Scotland in 1985, and seven areas of England and Scotland in 1987, had a co-ordinated approach involving the general public, GPs and dermatologists. The latter study was funded by the Cancer Research Campaign (CRC). Pigmented Lesion Clinics (PLCs) were set up in each study area to ensure a quick referral system to hospital, GPs were advised about the seven-point checklist and about referral to PLCs for which the patient did not need an appointment at all, but one clinic and a high profile health education programme targeted at the general public was then launched using the media, posters and leaflets.

A similar type of campaign has taken place in Italy [16]. In Australia, early detection has been promoted alongside extensive primary prevention initiatives but there appears to have been little evaluation of any early detection campaign. In a study of the general population in an area of New South Wales [24] 48% had their skin checked regularly by themselves or by another person and 17% had been screened by a GP in the previous 12 months. However, the effectiveness of these screening procedures was not assessed. In other campaigns in Europe [5, 9, 38, 57] various methods of publicity have been used such as house-to-house delivery of leaflets and television broadcasts but not all campaigns were linked with provision of health services and data collection as in the British studies.

Evaluation of Health Education Programmes

Ideally self-screening for melanoma should be evaluated in a randomised controlled trial but so far this has not taken place. The main difficulty with the evaluation of health education programmes is that it is virtually impossible to ensure that the control population remains unaffected by the health education messages particularly if the media publicise the campaign. In contrast to screening for breast or cervical cancer which requires sophisticated medical techniques and equipment operated by trained staff, clinical screening for melanoma can be attempted by anyone and as public awareness about the disease increases so too will self-screening.

The most important aim of early detection is to identify and treat cases which would otherwise progress to death and thus to reduce mortality from melanoma. A minimum of seven years follow-up would be required to evaluate the impact of a health education programme on mortality. In the interim other outcome measures can be studied: the impact of the programme on awareness about melanoma, on workload for the health services, characteristics of patients attending clinics, psychosocial and economic effects and trends in incidence of melanoma by stage or more commonly Breslow thickness which is strongly associated with prognosis.

Effect on Mortality

There is no conclusive evidence that health education campaigns have significantly reduced mortality from melanoma. In Scotland a decline in the mortality rate for melanoma in women, not men, following the 1985 Glasgow campaign was reported but there were several problems with the method of analysis [43]. The rates were reported for the whole of Scotland although the campaign focused on the West of

Scotland. Subsequently, results reported from South East Scotland show no decline in thick tumours during the same period [29]. There was no control population and as the rates are crude cross-sectional ones other factors could have influenced the change in rates besides the campaign. Thus overall the results from Scotland show some inconsistencies and at the very least may only benefit women. If this result is confirmed elsewhere it will be important to re-examine the health education methods to investigate whether screening can be made more effective for men. It is possible that health education may be less effective in this group because a high proportion of male melanomas are nodular and occur on the back.

In a much smaller study in Italy, a decline or levelling of mortality from melanoma was reported following a campaign similar to that in the UK. However, there are some inconsistencies in the pattern of mortality rates over time in both the study and neighbouring control areas and it may be difficult to show a significant result with a sample size of only 434 000 [17].

Finally, mortality rates for melanoma may be levelling off in some sections of the populations in the USA [62], Australia [6] and Sweden [68]. It is possible that increased awareness about the early signs of melanoma in the general population may have contributed to these trends. However, other environmental, social, behavioural or dietary changes could have taken place to have influenced the changes in mortality rates.

Effect on Stage-specific Incidence

Most early detection programmes for melanoma have been associated with increased reporting of melanomas with thin Breslow thickness < 0.76 mm. This has been found in the UK programmes [25, 43, 70], Italy [16] and Switzerland [9]. The incidence rates of thin tumours have also been rising rapidly in areas of Australia [6, 46]. However, the thin tumours are likely to include a proportion of non-progressive tumours and survival estimates based on the mean Breslow thickness and the percentage distribution of each case may be subject to lead time bias and length biased sampling. The most important trend to study is the incidence rate of thick tumours (Breslow thickness ≥ 3.5 mm). A decrease in incidence of thick melanomas is likely to be correlated with a later decline in mortality rate for melanoma.

The findings of several studies are summarised in Table 5.3. Positive results come from Scotland [43] and Italy [16]. In the former study over a period of five years, one year after the start of the campaign a significant decrease in the incidence rate of thick melanoma was reported for women, but not men. In Italy a decrease in incidence was also reported averaged over two four-year periods after the start of the campaign compared with a four-year period precampaign but this result was not compared with control areas or studied by sex. In contrast, in two of the British study areas no decrease in thick tumours was found over a five-year period following the 1987 campaign [27, 29]. In two other areas of the British study it was found that in the first year after the campaign a decline in thick tumours was consistent with a similar trend before the campaign [70, 71]. In a collaborative study of all seven study areas which participated in the CRC early detection programme no significant change was found for the incidence rate of melanomas with Breslow thickness ≥ 3.5 mm up to 2½ years after the intervention, and there was also no significant difference in this trend between areas [51].

Table 5.3 Summary of findings in programmes for the early detection of melanoma

Reference	Study area/country	Health education and screening process, and year of programme	Months of follow-up	Change in incidence of melanomas with thick Breslow thickness	Change in melanoma mortality
Whitehead et al. [70]	Nottingham, England	General public health education and referral via GPs to dermatologists, 1987	6 months	No change in distribution with precampaign period, Breslow > 3.5 mm	Evaluation of mortality underway in 7 CRC study areas
Williams et al. [71]	King's College Hospital, London, England	General public health education and referral via GPs to dermatologists, 1986	12 months	No change in distribution with precampaign period, Breslow > 3.5 mm	
Healsmith et al. [27]	Leicester, England	General public health education and referral via GPs to dermatologists, 1987	48 months	No change, Breslow ≥3.5 mm	
Herd et al. [29]	South-East Scotland	General public health education and referral via GPs to dermatologists, 1987	36 months	No change, Breslow ≥3.5 mm	
MacKie and Hole [43]	Scotland	General public health education and referral via GPs to dermatologists, 1985	48 months	Women: significant reduction, Breslow ≥3.5 mm. Men: no change	Possible reduction in women
MacKie and Hole [43]	Scotland	General public health education and referral via GPs to dermatologists, 1985	48 months		
Cristofolini et al. [16]	Trentino, Italy	General public health education, 1977	96 months	No change in incidence 1–4 years after campaign, but decrease 5–8 years later. Breslow ≥3 mm	
Cristofolini et al. [17]	Trentino, Italy	General public health education, 1977	96 months	No change, Breslow ≥3 mm	Cumulative mortality rates showed no change but less increase than in neighbouring areas
Bonerandi et al. [5]	1 region of France	General public health education via media, 1989	6 months	No change, Breslow > 3 mm	
Lejeune et al. [38]	Belgium	Information campaigns since 1983	48 months	Mean values of Breslow thickness showed no change over time	
Bulliard et al. [9]	Switzerland	General public self-screening, 1988	12 months	No consistent change in incidence over time, Breslow > 1.5 mm	
Pehamberger et al. [57]	Austria	General public health education, 1988 May–August 1988	36 months	No change in median or % distribution of Breslow > 3.0 mm	

No positive results have been reported from France [5] or Switzerland [9], but the follow-up periods in these studies were too short to have an impact on thick tumours. In Belgium, Lejeune et al. [38] reported no change in mean Breslow thickness in four years following their campaign but this is an insensitive measure of change. There is a similar problem with the results reported from Austria [57]. The median Breslow thickness and percentage distribution of Breslow thickness were used to demonstrate a possible benefit from an early detection campaign. However, both measures may be affected by lead-time and length bias if a proportion of early stage melanomas detected after the campaign were non-progressive. Results 2–3 years later showed no apparent difference in the distribution of thickness from that measured before the campaign.

Effect on Health Services Workload

The impact of early detection campaigns on the workload of general practitioners has been studied in the UK where campaigns have encouraged the general public to see their GPs about suspicious lesions [23, 25, 53, 70]. All reported an increase in GP workload. In Nottingham [70] the number of cases consulting with a discrete skin lesion per GP per week rose from 0.4 to 1.4. Similar increases were seen elsewhere. These numbers may seem small but they will still have an impact on workload especially since UK GPs have been encouraged to undertake skin biopsies. In a campaign in the Netherlands [58] in which the general public were invited to see the local dermatologist there was no impact on GP workload but this may be at the expense of excessive workload for the dermatologists.

Despite the benefit of involving GPs to screen out the least suspicious lesions, workload at dermatology clinics will increase dramatically after a campaign. In the British study there was overall a 6-fold increase in the number of referrals to the PLCs [25, 70] in the first two weeks immediately after the campaign which later settled down to a 2–4-fold increase [50].

The total number of referrals depended on the population size covered by the clinic and the extent to which GP referrals were sent to the PLCs rather than other hospital departments. In Nottingham, with a study population of 610 000 where most referrals went to the PLC, the average number of referrals per week initially rose to 54.8 and then settled down to 22.8. Approximately 27% of PLC referrals were then referred for biopsy so there was also considerable impact on pathology workload although this was not directly assessed [50]. The ratio of benign:malignant melanoma resulting from early detection campaigns has been reported. In Scotland [43] and England [50] ratios of 22:1 and 33:1, respectively, were reported which compares favourably with ratios of 253:1 at health fairs in the USA [3] and 256:1 in the Netherlands [58].

The final diagnosis is dependent on excisional biopsy and histological examination. Histological diagnosis can only be made with certainty if the lesion is completely excised. Because of the false positive errors in clinical diagnosis biopsies may be performed on a large proportion of benign lesions which is a disadvantage to patients, particularly if the lesions are in exposed sites such as the face. In addition the histological diagnosis is susceptible to error. Among borderline cases there is a risk of both over- and under-diagnosis. As very early stage lesions with Breslow thickness < 0.76 mm are unlikely to have metastasised, this cut-off point is often used in patient management, and only lesions with greater depth may require wider excision. However, the measurement of Breslow thickness is not completely reliable [15] and it is now proposed that the presence of the vertical growth phase in combination with other features may be a better marker for poor prognosis and thus patient management than Breslow thickness alone [13].

Organised Professional Screening

Screening for malignant melanoma by professional clinical examination has the advantages that it is non-invasive, safe, and requires no expensive or specialised equipment thus making it potentially accessible through GP and dermatological services. The disadvantages are that a thorough examination requires whole body examinations which may be unacceptable to some people [60], changes in a lesion are difficult for the patient or clinician to notice unless baseline photography is used, and thus a thorough screening procedure is very time consuming. Another important disadvantage of clinical examination is the errors in diagnosis which will cause both false positives and false negatives to occur even among dermatologists. Three main approaches have been studied: opportunistic professional screening at health fairs and walk-in clinics, screening in the workplace and screening of high risk groups.

Opportunistic Screening

Opportunistic professional screening has mainly been studied in the USA. As there is concern in the USA about legal liability from misdiagnosis, screening is usually conducted by dermatologists. Walk-in clinics and screening caravans have been set up in various settings. This approach was extended in 1985 to set up a series of free clinics in various parts of the country [35]. The American Academy of Dermatology (AAD) invited dermatologists to conduct annual free screenings for skin cancer. The AAD organised the publicity, distribution of education materials and encouraged use of a standardised recording form. The number of respondents had reached over 461 000 by 1991. Some assessments have been made of the individual clinics and these are now being evaluated together [35]. A similar approach to screening with free walk-in clinics has also been established in the Netherlands [58]. Although melanomas have been detected, the effectiveness of this method is dependent on the general public using the screening service, and complying with referral for further tests. The workload is high for a low yield of melanomas. Other skin conditions including non-melanomas may be detected but these usually have a good prognosis without early detection by screening [34]. In addition evaluation methods have not been standardised across all clinics and there is the problem of obtaining complete population based baseline data.

Screening at the Workplace

The advantages of screening at work are that, provided the employers co-operate to provide adequate facilities and time for the screening process, good response rates for both initial screening and follow-up can be obtained. However, the application of the approach to screening is limited and it is unlikely to have a major impact on the overall mortality from melanoma. In addition it may be difficult to ensure that screening programmes are run to similar standards across different work settings and organisations.

Screening of High-Risk Groups

The idea of identifying and screening high risk groups is an attractive one because melanomas will be detected more frequently than in the general population. The efficiency of this approach depends on the strength of the association between the risk factors and melanoma, and the proportion of all melanomas associated with the risk factors as well as the other aspects of screening such as the response rate and accuracy of the screening tests. People who carry a high risk of developing melanoma include those from families with the dysplastic naevus syndrome, and transplant and leukaemia patients [26, 37] but they will account for only a small proportion, perhaps less than 10%, of melanoma cases. Prevention of melanoma deaths in such cases will thus have little impact on the overall burden of disease.

Other risk factors have been proposed which may account for a higher proportion of cases [59]. In Scotland MacKie et al. [42] recommended a personal risk-factor chart using total number of pigmented naevi above 2 mm diameter, freckling tendency, number of clinically atypical naevi and history of severe sunburn to target prevention advice to those at greatest risk of the disease. However, the use of such a chart and its effect on prevalence at screening, stage and mortality, has not been evaluated. An alternative approach to identify populations at high risk would simply be to count naevi of a defined size on the arm, which correlates well with whole-body counts [65] and with those individuals who suffer mortality, ensuring that future campaigns target men and the elderly.

Evaluation of Professional Screening

Effect on Mortality

There have been no randomised controlled trials of professional screening for melanoma and thus there is no conclusive evidence that professional screening would help to reduce mortality from the disease.

In the USA professional screening was provided for employees of the Lawrence Livermore National Laboratory. Schneider et al [61] showed a reduction in mortality for melanoma from four fatalities in the prescreening period (9.0 per 100 000) to one fatality in the postscreening period (2.7 per 100 000). However, the trend was not compared with a control population. The screening was likely to have been far more intensive than that which would be practical on a large scale so even if the screening programme did benefit health its application to large populations is limited.

Effect on Stage-specific Incidence

For professional screening there is evidence of an increase in the proportion of early stage or thin melanoma either over time or compared with other populations [35]. However, evaluation is limited by lack of adequate control populations and by self-selection among the study population.

The effect of screening in the workplace on stage-specific incidence of melanoma has been reported from the Lawrence Livermore Laboratory study [61]. A decrease in the incidence of thick tumours (>5mm) was found following the provision of health education and free screening.

The effects of screening high risk groups on detection of melanomas by Breslow thickness has been investigated in several studies. Masri et al. [48] in the USA found that the Breslow thickness of newly detected melanomas in high risk families under group surveillance was significantly lower than for the index cases which had led to the surveillance of their relatives. MacKie et al. [45] reported a high detection rate of melanoma in patients classified according to a previous history of melanoma and/or atypical naevi, and provided with intensive screening which involved examination and photography every 3–6months. However, no comparison of self-screening with professional screening for high risk groups seems to have been made and further evaluation should be encouraged.

Other Aspects of Screening

Other effects of screening have not been fully explored. For all who are screened there could be anxiety associated with the screening examination and, among those receiving a biopsy or wider excision, the psychosocial effects of scarring, particularly in exposed places such as the face, have not been studied. True positives will experience social and psychological effects of being diagnosed with melanoma and the consequences related to employment and insurance. Errors in the screening test will lead to false negatives being falsely reassured and false positives undergoing unnecessary biopsies. There are resource costs to the health service in providing a service which will include unnecessary biopsies as well as personal costs to the individual. One possible additional advantage from screening is the detection of other treatable skin cancers or skin conditions which would otherwise in the long-term cause morbidity.

Before screening for melanoma is more widely promoted the cost-effectiveness needs to be studied. This aspect of screening is discussed in Chapter 10. Also, the frequency of screening has not yet been evaluated for the general population or high risk groups. The rate at which interval cancers present needs to be studied within a screening study.

Conclusions

There is no conclusive evidence that screening for melanoma in the general population has reduced mortality. However, this does not mean that a carefully organised programme, which ensures effective targeting of the study population, trained screening and thorough follow-up procedures, is ineffective. Although evaluation is still underway for studies of health education in the UK and abroad, it is essential that all future programmes are conducted as research trials with advanced planning and evaluation. Elwood [22] has proposed various options for randomised controlled trials of self-screening and screening by health professionals such as GPs. Detailed evaluation programmes would need to be set up to study all aspects of the screening process including uptake, frequency of screening, workload and effects on stage-specific incidence and mortality.

Various working groups and consensus panels have reviewed current knowledge about early detection for melanoma and their conclusions are mixed. Large scale screening of the general population was not supported by the International Union Against Cancer [32]. The US Preventive Sevices Task Force [69] and Canadian Task Force [10] only recommended screening for high risk groups. The American Cancer Society [2] recommended a physical examination of the skin every three years for 20–40-year-olds and annually for > 40-year-olds. The NIH Consensus Development Panel [54] in the USA supported screening but the recommendations are based on the results of the health education programme in Scotland alone referred to above. The American Cancer Society [2] and American Academy of Dermatology [1] and National Cancer Institute [52] recommend self-screening. However, reviews by several researchers [22, 35, 47] point to the importance of evaluation in all future work. Awareness about melanoma will increase in the general population whether or not specific campaigns are launched because primary prevention programmes are bound to stimulate public concern about skin cancer. Therefore, it is important that health services should be prepared for an increase in workload, ensure optimum practice in the handling, reporting and referral of suspect lesions and that there should be high quality cancer registration with which to monitor trends in incidence by Breslow thickness and mortality.

References

1. American Academy of Dermatology (1992) Summary report of the AAD Committee on Melanoma/Skin Cancer Screening Program. Schaumburg, Illinois.
2. American Cancer Society (1980) Report on cancer-related health check-up. CA 30:194–240.
3. Arundell FD (1986) Screening for melanoma and skin cancer. JAMA 255:2443–2444.
4. Bergman W, Fusero RM (1992) Precursor lesions to melanoma. Clin Dermatol 10:21–29.
5. Bonerandi JJ, Grob JJ, Cnudde N et al. (1992) Campagne de détéction, précoce du mélanome dans la région Provence–Alps–Côte D'Azur–Corse en 1989. Ann Dermatol

Venereol 119:105–109.

6. Bonett A, Roder D, Esterman A (1989) Epidemiological features of melanoma in South Australia: implications for cancer control. Med J Aust 151:502–509.

7. Borland R, Marks R, Noy S (1992) Public knowledge about characteristics of moles and melanomas. Aust J Public Health 16:370–375.

8. Breslow A (1970) Thickness, cross-sectional area and depth of invasion in the prognosis of cutaneous melanoma. Ann Surg 172:902–908.

9. Bulliard J-L, Raymond L, Levi F, et al. (1992) Prevention of cutaneous melanoma: an epidemiological evaluation of the Swiss campaign. Rev Epidemiol Santé Publique 40:431–438.

10. Canadian Task Force on the Periodic Health Examination (1984) The periodic health examination: 2. 1984 update. Can Med Assoc J 130:1278–1285.

11. Cannon-Albright LA, Goldger DE, Meyer LJ et al. (1992) Assignment of a locus for familial melanoma, MLM, to chromosome 9p13–p22. Science 258:1148–1152.

12. Cassileth BR, Clark WH Jr, Heiberger RM et al. (1982) Relationship between patients' early recognition of melanoma and depth of invasion. Cancer 49:198–200.

13. Clark WH Jr, Elder DE, Guerry IV D et al. (1989) Model predicting survival in Stage I melanoma based on tumour progression. J Natl Cancer Inst 81(21):1893–1904.

14. Coleman M, Esteve J, Damiecke P (1993) Trends in cancer incidence and mortality. IARC, no. 121. Lyon.

15. Colloby PS, West KP, Fletcher A (1991) Observer variation in the measurement of Breslow depth and Clark's level in thin cutaneous malignant melanoma. J Pathol 163:245–250.

16. Cristofolini M, Zumiani G, Boi S, Piscioli F (1986) Community detection of early melanoma. Lancet i:156.

17. Cristofolini M, Bianchi R, Boi S et al. (1993) Effectiveness of the health campaign for the early diagnosis of cutaneous melanoma in Trentino, Italy. J Dermatol Surg Oncol 19:117–120.

18. du Vivier AWP, Williams HC, Brett JV, Higgins EM (1991) How do malignant melanomas present and does this correlate with the seven-point check-list? Clin Exp Dermatol 16:344–347.

19. Dunkley MP, Morris AM (1991) Cutaneous malignant melanoma: audit of the diagnostic process. Ann R Coll Surg Eng 73:248–252.

20. Ellman R (1991) Screening for melanoma in the UK. In: Miller AB, Chamberlain J, Day NE, Hakama M, Prorok PC (eds) Cancer screening. UICC project on evaluation of screening for cancer. Cambridge University Press, Cambridge, pp 257–266.

21. Elwood JM (1992) Melanoma and ultraviolet radiation. Clin Dermatol 10:41–50.

22. Elwood JM (1994) Screening for melanoma and options for its evaluation. J Med Screening 1:22–38.

23. Farris GM (1988) The effect of the 1987 melanoma campaign on the workload of general practitioners and dermatologists. Br J Dermatol 119(Suppl):24.

24. Girgis A, Campbell EM, Redman S et al. (1991) Screening for melanoma: a community survey of prevalence and predictors. Med J Aust 154:338–343.

25. Graham-Brown RAC, Osborne JE, London SP et al. (1990) The initial effects on workload and outcome of a public education campaign on early diagnosis and treatment of malignant melanoma in Leicestershire. Br J Dermatol 122:53–59.

26. Green A, Smith P, McWhirter W et al. (1993) Melanocytic naevi and melanoma in survivors of childhood cancer. Br J Cancer 67:1053–1057.

27. Healsmith MF, Graham-Brown RAC, Osborne JC et al. (1993) Further experience of

public education for the early diagnosis of malignant melanoma in Leicestershire. Clin Exp Dermatol 18:396–400.

28. Hennrikus D, Girgis A, Redman S et al. (1991) A community study of delay in presenting with signs of melanoma to medical practitioners. Arch Dermatol 127:356–361.

29. Herd RM, Cooper EJ, Hunter JAA et al. (1995) Cutaneous malignant melanoma. Publicity, screening clinics and survival – the Edinburgh experience 1982–1990. Br J Dermatol 132:563–570.

30. Higgins EM, Hall P, Todd P et al. (1992) The application of the seven-point check-list in the assessment of benign pigmented lesions. Clin Exp Dermatol 17:313–315.

31. Holman CDJ, Armstrong BK (1984) Pigmentary traits, ethnic origin, benign nevi, and family history as risk factors for cutaneous malignant melanoma. J Natl Cancer Inst 72:257–266.

32. International Union Against Cancer (UICC) (1992) Melanoma control manual, UICC, Geneva.

33. Keefe M, Dick DC, Wakeel RA (1990) A study of the value of the seven-point checklist in distinguishing benign pigmented lesions from melanoma. Clin Exp Dermatol 15:167–171.

34. Koh HK, Caruso A, Gage I et al. (1990) Evaluation of melanoma/skin cancer screening in Massachusetts. Cancer 65:375–379.

35. Koh HK, Geller AC, Miller DR et al. (1993) Early detection of melanoma: an ounce of prevention may be a ton of work. J Am Acad Dermatol 28:645–647.

36. Koh HK, Miller DR, Geller AC et al. (1992) Who discovers melanoma? J Am Acad Dermatol 26:914–919.

37. Kraemer KH, Greene MH, Tarone R et al. (1983) Dysplastic naevi and cutaneous melanoma risk. Lancet ii:1076–1077.

38. Lejeune FJ, Lienard D, Andre J (1991) Malignant melanoma: an epidemiological phenomenon. Dev Oncol 63:125–138.

39. McGovern TW, Litaker MS (1992) Clinical predictors of malignant pigmented lesions. A comparison of the Glasgow seven-point checklist and the American Cancer Society's ABCDs of pigmented lesions. J Dermatol Surg Oncol 18:22–26.

40. MacKie RM (1986) An illustrated guide to the recognition of early malignant melanoma. University of Glasgow, Glasgow.

41. MacKie RM (1990) Clinical recognition of early invasive malignant melanoma. Br Med J 301:1005–1006.

42. MacKie RM, Freudenberger T, Aitchison TC (1989) Personal risk-factor chart for cutaneous melanoma. Lancet ii:487–490.

43. MacKie RM, Hole D (1992) Audit of public education campaign to encourage earlier detection of malignant melanoma. Br Med J 304:1012–1015.

44. Mackie RM, Hunter JAA, Aitchison TC et al. (1992) Cutaneous malignant melanoma, Scotland, 1979–89. Lancet 339:971–975.

45. MacKie RM, McHenry P, Hole D (1993) Accelerated detection with prospective surveillance for cutaneous malignant melanoma in high-risk groups. Lancet 341:1618–1620.

46. MacLennan R, Green AC, McLeod GRC, Martin NG (1992) Increasing incidence of cutaneous melanoma in Queensland, Australia. J Natl Cancer Inst 84(18):1427–1433.

47. Marks R, Hill D (1992) The public health approach to melanoma control. Prevention and early detection. Melbourne: UICC, Australian Cancer Society.

48. Masri GD, Clark WH, Guerry D et al. (1990) Screening and surveillance of patients at

high risk for malignant melanoma result in detection of earlier disease. J Am Acad Dermatol 22:1042–1048.

49. Melia J, Ellman R, Chamberlain J (1994) Investigating changes in awareness about cutaneous malignant melanoma in Britain using the Omnibus Survey. Clin Exp Dermatol 19:375–379.

50. Melia J, Cooper EJ, Frost T et al. (1995) Cancer Research Campaign Health Education Programme to promote the early detection of cutaneous malignant melanoma I. Workload and referral patterns. Br J Dermatol 132:405–413.

51. Melia J, Cooper EJ, Frost T et al. (1995) Cancer Research Campaign Health Education Programme to promote the early detection of cutaneous malignant melanoma II. Characteristics and incidence of melanoma. Br J Dermatol 132:414–421.

52. National Cancer Institute (1987) Working guidelines for early cancer detection: rationale and supporting evidence to decrease mortality. National Cancer Institute, Bethesda, Maryland.

53. Nichols S (1988) Effect of a public campaign about malignant melanoma on general practitioner workload in Southampton. Br Med J 296:1526.

54. NIH Consensus Development Panel on Early Melanoma (1992) Diagnosis and treatment of early melanoma. JAMA 268:1314–1319.

55. Office of Population Censuses and Surveys (1993) 1987 Cancer statistics registrations. Series MBI No. 20. HMSO, London.

56. Office of Population Censuses and Surveys (1993) 1992 Mortality statistics cause. Series DH2 No. 19. HMSO, London.

57. Pehamberger H, Binder M, Knollmayer S, Wolff K (1993) Immediate effects of a public education campaign on prognostic features of melanoma. J Am Acad Dermatol 29:106–109.

58. Rampen FH, Berretty PJM, van Huystee BEWL (1993) General practitioners' workload after skin cancer/melanoma screening clinics in the Netherlands. Dermatology 186: 258–260.

59. Rhodes AR, Weinstock MA, Fitzpatrick TB et al. (1987) Risk factors for cutaneous melanoma. A practical method of recognizing predisposed individuals. JAMA 258:3146–3154.

60. Rigel DS, Friedman RJ, Kopf AW et al. (1986) Importance of complete cutaneous examination for the detection of malignant melanoma. J Am Acad Dermatol 15:857–860.

61. Schneider JS, Sagebiel RW, Moore II DH, Lawton GM (1987) Melanoma surveillance and earlier diagnosis. Lancet i:1435.

62. Scotto J, Pitcher H, Lee JAH (1991) Indications of future decreasing trends in skin-melanoma among whites in the United States. Int J Cancer 49:490–497.

63. Shaw HM, McCarthy WH (1992) Small-diameter malignant melanoma: a common diagnosis in New South Wales, Australia. J Acad Dermatol 27:679–682.

64. Southampton Melanoma Group (1986) Effects of rapid referral on thickness of melanoma. Br Med J 293:790.

65. Swerdlow AJ, English J, MacKie RM et al. (1984) Benign naevi associated with a high risk factor of melanoma. Lancet ii:168.

66. Swerdlow AJ, English J, MacKie RM et al. (1986) Benign melanocytic naevi: as a risk factor for malignant melanoma. Br Med J 292:1555–1559.

67. Temoshok L, DiClemente R, Sweet D, Blois M, Sagabiel R (1984) Factors relating to delay in seeking medical attention for cutaneous malignant melanoma. Cancer 54: 3048–3053.

68. Thorn M, Sparen P, Bergstrom R et al. (1992) Trends in mortality rates from malignant melanoma in Sweden 1953–1987 and forecasts up to 2007. Br J Cancer 66:563–567.
69. United States Preventive Services Task Force (1992) Guide to clinical preventive services: an assessment of the effectiveness of 169 interventions. Williams and Wilkins, Baltimore.
70. Whitehead SM, Wroughton MA, Elwood JM, Davison J, Stewart M (1989) Effects of a health education campaign for the earlier diagnosis of melanoma. Br J Cancer 60:421–425.
71. Williams HC, Smith D, du Vivier AWP (1990) Evaluation of public education campaigns in cutaneous melanoma: the King's College Hospital experience. Br J Dermatol 123:85–92.

6 – Screening for Ovarian Cancer

Howard Cuckle

Introduction

Ovarian cancer is the most common gynaecological malignancy in developed countries, with about twice the incidence of cervical cancer. Two features of the disease which are relevant to screening are the much longer survival when the disease is confined to the ovary compared to more advanced presentations and the fact that most cases present clinically with symptoms due to advanced disease. The International Federation of Gynaecology and Obstetrics (FIGO) have collected data from several countries on over 8000 ovarian cancer cases classified using a standardised staging system [27]. Table 6.1 shows the 5-year survival rates according to stage and the proportion of cases presenting at the different stages. There was a 17-fold range in 5-year survival rates between tumours diagnosed when confined to a single ovary (Stage Ia) and those with distant metastases (Stage IV); less than one-fifth presented with a tumour confined to one or both ovaries (Stages Ia or Ib). Any screening test that would lead to considerably more cases being diagnosed at stage Ia or Ib would, therefore, seem to offer the opportunity of improving prognosis unless the observed differences in survival are entirely due to lead time and length bias. Although several protocols have been described, based on the use of one or more tests, their efficacy remains to be established in a study which avoids bias. In this chapter the component tests and the protocols are assessed. Although definitive studies have not yet been carried out, the results of preliminary investigations and feasibility studies have been published.

General Requirements

The central issue in ovarian cancer screening is whether there are protocols good enough to achieve a worthwhile reduction in mortality. Ultimately that can only be established by a clinical trial in which an extremely large number of asymptomatic women are randomly assigned either to be screened or to act as a control group. Screening would need to be repeated at regular intervals and the population followed-up for several years. However, given the large scale of such a trial there would have to be strong evidence that a specific protocol is likely to be of benefit before it was undertaken. Preliminary experience with the screening test will be required so that its performance and practicability can be judged.

Table 6.1   Five-year survival rate according to stage

Stage	Description	Cases	Survival (%)
Ia	Confined to one ovary[a]	1281	79.3
Ib	Confined to both ovaries	295	71.2
Ic	Not confined to the ovary	657	60.7
IIa	Extension or metastases to uterus or tubes	272	51.8
IIb & c	Further extension in pelvis	1043	44.8
III	Extension to abdomen	3371	18.4
IV	Distant metastases	1422	4.7
Overall		8341	35.0

Based on cases reported to the International Federation of Gynaecology and Obstetrics which could be staged [27].

[a] i.e. there are no ascites, the tumour is not on the external surface and the capsule is intact.

Size of Trial

Even on fairly optimistic assumptions the number of women randomised would be extremely large. If we assume that (a) screening begins at age 50 years, (b) it transfers two-thirds of those who would have presented with advanced disease to a localised stage, (c) the mortality rate in the additional women with an early diagnosis is similar to that in those presenting clinically at that stage, and (d) 75% of those offered randomisation agree, then 150 000 women would be needed. If followed-up for seven years a population of this size in the UK would yield an expected 66 deaths in the arm offered screening compared with 99 in the control arm. Such a trial would have 80% power to establish this level of benefit at the 5% level of significance.

Performance

So far a randomised trial of ovarian cancer screening with mortality as the endpoint has not been undertaken although interest has been expressed in various protocols. When considering which of them, if any, performs well enough to be subjected to the full rigours of a trial, the principal indices will be sensitivity and specificity.

With ovarian cancer the information on sensitivity mainly derives from studies carried out in women who were being investigated prior to diagnostic surgery. These retrospective studies are likely to introduce bias: any association between the average level of the test variable and clinical stage will lead to an exaggeration of performance. Prospective studies in asymptomatic women would yield more realistic estimates of sensitivity but they too have their limitations. In general the period of follow-up will be small and the number of malignancies expected in a given study will not be large enough to reliably assess sensitivity. Specificity can be more readily estimated. Since ovarian cancer is relatively rare the distribution of test results in any series of asymptomatic women will approximate to that in the unaffected population.

Practicability

There is no reason to expect that any of the tests being suggested for ovarian cancer screening will, of themselves, be unacceptable to women. They are no more invasive or uncomfortable than those used in screening programmes for breast and cervix cancer. Since the latter have reasonably high uptake it is likely that the ovarian cancer screening may also be generally acceptable.

There is, however, a major practical disadvantage to ovarian cancer screening not shared by the other malignancies, namely a low positive predictive value. When ovarian cancer is suspected clinically a confident diagnosis of malignancy will rest on the results of laparotomy. The procedure is expensive and hazardous but in symptomatic patients that is acceptable given the need to respond to symptoms and because of the high prior probability of abdominal malignancy. The situation is different when screening asymptomatic women is being proposed. A putative ovarian cancer screening test would need to have high specificity in order to select women for laparotomy who are at sufficiently great risk of cancer to justify the surgery (i.e. high positive predictive value). Even if the average lead time were 3 years a woman screened at age 50 years using a test with 95% specificity and 100% sensitivity the risk would only be 1 in 60.

The extent of the problem is dependent on the way in which benign masses and tumour-like conditions such as teratoma and endometrioma are dealt with. All of the tests being considered will to some extent lead to the incidental detection of these lesions. Some would regard the finding and removal of non-malignant ovarian or adnexal lesions as a benefit of screening. Firstly, many of them will eventually lead to medical problems (e.g. torsion) and early non-emergency removal would be an advantage. Secondly, if benign tumours were precursors of malignancy with a high rate of progression then their early treatment may be preventive. However, the early natural history of ovarian cancer is not well enough understood to be certain of this [1, 29].

If a less invasive means of making a diagnosis could replace laparotomy for lesions detected by screening the problem might not be so serious. Some benign conditions can be identified using laparoscopy but many malignant tumours, especially those diagnosed at an a early stage, can have a normal appearance. Also the procedure has a high complication rate [15] and therefore may have little advantage over laparotomy. Neither is fine needle aspiration a reliable alternative. In one series of 59 cysts aspirated prior to laparotomy, only two of seven cancers were identified and one of 52 benign cysts was wrongly classified as malignant [21].

On balance, it would be prudent to regard the incidental diagnosis of a benign lesion as a false-positive result. In which case, specificity will need to be considerably in excess of 95%.

Candidate Tests: Evidence from Observational Studies

The only tests which are remotely sensitive enough to be considered for use in ovarian cancer screening are tumour markers in blood or urine and ultrasound. Physical examination, although widely practised in well women's clinics, is insensitive.

Tumour Markers

Ovarian tumours are associated with the increased production or altered metabolism of various chemicals which results in raised blood or urine levels (see [20] and [65] for a review). Some of the markers are strong enough determinants of the presence of tumour cells to be of value in clinical practice by aiding diagnosis and in monitoring relapse after initial treatment. To be useful in patient follow-up a marker needs to be sensitive. Sequential testing at short intervals with a sensitive marker may reveal the presence of recurrence before it is clinically apparent and obviate the need for second look laparoscopy. None the less it does not mean that such a marker would be sensitive enough for screening asymptomatic women. This can be readily demonstrated for CA 125, a widely used tumour marker in clinical practice and the only one that has been examined in a screening context.

CA 125

This marker was developed by raising a monoclonal antibody in an ovarian cancer cell line [7]. The antibody reacts with a cell surface antigen on most histological types of non-mucinous epithelial ovarian tumours. In women who present clinically with ovarian cancer, serum CA 125 levels are elevated above 35 U/ml in over 80% of cases whereas less than 5% of unaffected women have such an elevation (for a review see [18] and [37]). Although sensitivity appears to be slightly lower in mucinous tumours it is largely unrelated to histological type. Overall sensitivity is reasonably high but there is a clear correlation between the CA 125 level and the clinical stage of the disease indicating that sensitivity will be lower in less-advanced tumours. Thus under 50% of those presenting with FIGO Stage I disease have raised levels compared with over 90% in those with Stage IV. Moreover, the sensitivity in asymptomatic women has been shown to be even lower. This finding is from the JANUS study, based on a prospectively collected and stored serum bank from apparently healthy individuals [78]. Samples were retrieved and tested for CA 125 after ovarian cancer had presented clinically in 105 women up to 12 years after blood was taken. Levels were raised above 35 U/ml in only 17% and those with the highest levels tended to present clinically within a relatively short period after blood being taken. Table 6.2 shows the trend in detection rate according to the lead time in the JANUS study and the clinical stage among symptomatic patients. These results suggest that CA 125 would be an insensitive screening test for cases of ovarian cancer which were at a treatable stage.

Table 6.2 CA 125: proportion with raised levels according to the lead time in the JANUS study and the stage at diagnosis in symtomatic patients

	Cases	CA 125 ≥ 35 U/ml
JANUS study [78]		
> 3 years[a]	77	11 (14%)
1–3 years	20	4 (20%)
< 1 year	8	3 (38%)
Symptomatic patients [18]		
Stage I[b]	128	56 (44%)
Stage II	59	52 (88%)
Stage III	275	250 (91%)
Stage IV	106	100 (94%)

[a]Time between blood being taken and the clinical diagnosis.
[b]FIGO classification.

Serum CA 125 levels tend to be raised in the presence of benign disease of the reproductive and digestive tracts, as well as with cancers at various sites [37]. A significant proportion of women have raised levels in the following conditions: benign ovarian tumour (about 10%), endometriosis (20%–30%), liver cirrhosis (60%–70%), pancreatitis (30%), or cancer of the endometrium (30%), lung (30%), stomach (30%), pancreas (50%) and liver (50%). Screening for ovarian cancer will therefore lead to the incidental diagnosis of some of these disorders, possibly leading to overtreatment.

Other Markers

Antigenic markers other than CA 125 have been reported to be raised in the presence of ovarian cancer as have oncofetal proteins and other tumour associated chemicals. Table 6.3 shows the results for 15 markers using studies in which a direct comparison can be made between the alternative marker and CA 125 on the same samples. In each of the studies the cut-off level for the two markers being compared had been chosen so as to yield similar specificity. The markers that have been most often been compared with CA 125 have a lower sensitivity; there are markers (for example urinary gonadotropin fragment) which might have higher sensitivity than CA 125 but they have not yet been examined in sufficient series to be sure of this. All of these results relate to clinically presenting cases, and it is unlikely that an alternative marker would be better than CA 125 at detecting early tumours, and it might even be worse with more advanced disease.

Ultrasound

An ultrasound examination can be used to determine whether the ovary is enlarged, has abnormal morphology or the blood flow to it is altered. The scan may be performed with either an abdominal or vaginal transducer. The transvaginal route has the advantage that a full bladder is not required and it produces a more precise image because of the proximity of the ovary.

Table 6.3   Sensitivity of alternative markers compared with that of CA 125

Alternative marker[a]	Study reference number	Cases	Sensitivity (%)	
			CA 125	Alternative
TAG	[31]	34	88	65
	[60]	44	86	66
	[8]	47	91	49
	[53]	106	81	62
CA 19–9	[31]	34	88	21
	[52]	119	90	36
CA 15–3	[8]	47	91	57
	[77]	50	72	56
CA M29	[77]	50	72	60
	[23]	92	75	67
HMFG–2	[8]	47	91	62
	[25]	215	80	60
HMFG–1	[8]	47	91	77
CA 54/61	[66]	40	88	60
CA M26	[77]	50	72	32
CA 130	[45]	126	90	91
CA 125II	[43]	46	91	98
NB/70K	[8]	47	91	57
LSA	[61]	89	76	71
UGF	[16]	71	70	82
PLAP	[8]	47	91	25
MCF	[76]	69	64	68

[a]TAG = tumour associated glycoprotein; HMFG = human milk fat globule; LSA = lipid associated sialic acid; UGF = urinary gonadotropin fragment; PLAP = placental alkaline phosphatase; MCF = macrophage colony-stimulating factor.

Size

Ultrasound is capable of identifying changes in ovarian size that would be apparent before the ovary became palpable. This can be quantified by either the maximum diameter of the ovary or its volume. Ovarian shape approximately corresponds to an ellipsoid, so that a simple geometric formula can be used to estimate volume from the largest three orthogonal diameters. The definition of ovarian enlargement is made by comparing the measured diameter or volume with the normal range or with the size of the contralateral ovary.

Ovarian abnormality is clearly associated with enlargement. In one study 52 postmenopausal women referred for reasons other than an adnexal mass had trans-vaginal ultrasound prior to surgery [56]. Ten ovaries were found to have some abnormality and nine of them had a diameter exceeding 2 cm. By comparison, of 94 normal ovaries, all were under 3 cm with an average diameter of 1 cm.

Observational studies which report ovarian size cannot be used to judge the likely screening sensitivity and specificity as they include a disproportionate number of women referred for ultrasound with a palpable pelvic mass. They do, however, provide an indication that ovaries containing malignant masses are larger than benign ones. In one study of 120 women with benign or malignant ovarian masses all but one of 41 with malignancy had a diameter exceeding 5 cm compared with 73% (58/79) among those with benign tumours or cysts [57]. In two similar studies the proportions were 100% (18/18) and 55% (28/51), respectively, in the first [50] with 60% (6/10) and 37% (71/190) in the second [59].

Morphology

A normal ovary should display a smooth outline and have a uniform low level echogenicity similar to that of the myometrium. Abnormality may be indicated by the presence of a mass, by its outline, location, locularity, contents and complexity and by the presence of ascites. As with ovarian size, observational studies tend to be carried out in women who already have a mass. Consequently they cannot readily be used to assess the potential screening sensitivity and specificity but they can indicate the value of assessing morphology once an enlarged ovary has been found in order to distinguish benign from malignant lesions.

In the past, the definition of abnormal morphology has not been consistent across studies. Moreover size as well as appearance will have been taken into account when interpreting the results. This has made it difficult to combine published results in a manner which would help predict performance. Given these limitations the available data from published studies on ultrasound carried out prior to surgery suggest that it does have reasonable discriminatory value. For example, in seven series combined, 77% of those confirmed to have ovarian cancer had abnormal scans compared with only 6% in those without cancer [18].

Various systems have been suggested whereby the complexity of morphological features is combined into a simple reproducible index of malignancy. If widely adopted that might allow a better comparison to be made between centres. Using a system to assign a grade of either 0, 1 or 2, in one study 54% (42/78) of malignancies had grade 2 and a further 23% (18/78) had grade 1, whereas the corresponding proportions among 399 benign cysts and tumours were 2% and 6% respectively [67]. Systems have also been described which yield a score in the range 1–10 [9, 24] or 4–15 (based on the addition of scores for each of four different features) [59].

Blood flow

Doppler ultrasound flow imaging is used to identify neovascularisation, a common concomitant of cancer [28]. Unlike standard ultrasound a computer generated image is produced with artificial colour to indicate the presence and direction of any blood flow within the tumour. If there is colour in the image this will be interpreted according to the visual appearance of the blood vessels and by two quantitative indices. An electronic gate is placed across the locus of interest to measure the Doppler shift. The measurements are used to compute the pulsatility index (peak systolic minus end diastolic flow divided by mean velocity) and the resistance index (systolic minus diastolic divided by systolic). New blood vessels with their elastic walls will have lower resistance to blood flow than well established vessels and hence lower values for both indices.

Table 6.4 shows the results of seven studies in which colour flow imaging was carried out prior to surgery in women with an ovarian mass. There was little overlap in the distribution of flow values between malignant and benign masses except for the Izumo research group which had previously reported encouraging results using Doppler but without colour [33]. These studies are encouraging and although not directly applicable to the use of Doppler in the primary screen they do suggest that it might be a useful secondary procedure in women found at screening to have enlarged ovaries. Furthermore, the secondary detailed scan could take account of both morphology and blood flow. In the Doppler study from New York [68] morphology was assessed using a standard scoring system [59]. All 16 malignancies could be identified by having either a high score or low flow whereas all 78 benign masses had a low score and high flow.

Table 6.4 Colour flow imaging prior to surgery: the results of seven studies of women with ovarian masses

Study	Index	Cut-off	Reduced flow	
			Malignant	Benign
Zagreb [48]	Resistance	0.50	100% (10/10)	0% (0/32)
London [11]	Pulsatility	1.00	88% (7/8)	10% (1/10)
Izumo [34]	Resistance	0.72	93% (25/27)	47% (17/36)
Nashville [26]	Pulsatility	1.00	100% (5/5)	14% (3/21)
Haifa [71]	Pulsatility	1.00	94% (16/17)	3% (1/36)
Nagoya [42]	Pulsatility	1.25	89% (8/9)	0% (0/15)
New York [68]	Resistance	0.46	95% (15/16)	1% (1/78)
	Pulsatility	0.62	88% (14/16)	3% (2/78)

The distinction between benign and malignant masses detected at screening might be further advanced by the use of computed tomography [58], magnetic resonance imaging [6, 34, 36] or immunoscintigraphy [64].

Improving Performance

Information derived from the observational series suggests that the currently available techniques may be inadequate for use in a screening context. For a suitable screening protocol, requiring high positive predictive value, it may be necessary to optimise the test for use in screening, to combine information on more than one test and to target more precisely the population which is invited for screening.

Optimising a Test

Altering the Cut-off Level

An improvement in specificity can usually be obtained by changing the cut-off level used to define a quantitative test result. With a qualitative test this is equivalent to raising the threshold of suspicion when interpreting the result. However, the gain in specificity will inevitably be at the cost of reduced sensitivity. For example, raising the CA 125 cut-off from 35 U/ml to 65 U/ml in the JANUS study increased specificity from 94.5% to 99.1% while reducing sensitivity from 17% to 6% [78].

Reducing Variability

By identifying the sources of normal variability, and where possible reducing their influence, the discriminatory power of the test can be improved. This has been attempted both for CA 125 and ultrasound by taking account of age and menopausal status.

Age   The level of CA 125 decreases on average with age. For example, in one study of 1802 women the proportion with levels exceeding 35 U/ml was 5% for the 483 aged 40–49 years, 3% for the 376 aged 50–59 years and 1% for the 223 aged 60 years or more [79]. Similarly, ovarian size also decreases with age [3, 14]. If age-specific cut-off levels were chosen such that the false-positive rate at each age was the same as the overall rate using a fixed cut-off, then the sensitivity would be increased.

Since the incidence of ovarian cancer varies according to age the optimal strategy would be to estimate for each woman the risk of having ovarian cancer given her age and test value. The risk would then be used as a composite screening variable reflecting both the probability of disease prior to testing and the test result. If the risk exceeded a given cut-off the result would be regarded as positive. A similar method has been used successfully in antenatal screening for Down's syndrome [19].

Menopause   The level of CA 125 is on average lower in postmenopausal women than before the menopause [79]. This effect is additional to the steady reduction in levels with advancing age. Similarly ovarian volume in postmenopausal women is lower than in premenopausal women of the same age, gradually declining with the time interval since the last menstrual period [32]. Thus the adoption of cut-off levels appropriate for both menopausal status and age will further improve the discriminatory power of the test.

Ovulation is a complicating factor when using ultrasound to screen premenopausal women due to the presence of normal ovarian follicles or corpus luteal cysts. When ovarian enlargement is found it may be necessary to repeat the scan to determine if cyclical changes could account for the abnormality. Moreover the impedance to blood flow in an ovulating ovary is similar to that in ovarian cancer. Therefore colour Doppler can yield falsely positive results.

Repeat Testing

Routinely repeating all tests and taking the average of the initial and repeat values reduces by half the components of variability such as assay imprecision and within-person fluctuations. If these represent a large fraction of total variability then discriminatory power may be substantially improved. However, even in these circumstances selective rather than routine repeat testing may be preferred for practical reasons. In general, restricting repeat testing to those with a positive initial test and using the repeat result in place of the original one will tend to have a dramatic effect on the false-positive rate. The increased specificity is, however, also likely to be accompanied by a reduction in sensitivity due to "regression to the mean". With progressive diseases like ovarian cancer where the mean value may become more extreme over time the loss of detection should not be great and the effect can be ameliorated by allowing for the original result when interpreting the repeat value.

Selective repeat testing has been investigated for CA 125 [79]. A total of 36 women with levels raised above 35 U/ml were retested sequentially at 3-monthly intervals. The average level fell by about one-third between the initial test and the first repeat test. In contrast the one case of ovarian cancer in the study group demonstrated rapidly rising levels from 35 U/ml at the first visit to 65 U/ml at 3 months and 206 U/ml at a year. The ultrasound findings were normal but a Stage III tumour was diagnosed at laparotomy 9 months later. Only one other woman had a large increase in CA 125 compared with the initial level and this was not sustained.

Combining Tests

The use of more than one test in screening can achieve better discrimination between affected and unaffected individuals than use of a single test. This is so even when the results of the component tests show a degree of correlation. Tests can be performed either sequentially or concurrently. In the former approach all women have a primary screening test and only those with abnormal results are offered another test or tests. As with repeat testing, specificity would be increased if both the primary and secondary screening test results had to be abnormal before the result was regarded as positive. However, sensitivity would also be decreased unless those with borderline results were also subjected to the second test.

With concurrent testing more than one test is performed on all women. Sensitivity would be increased if the result were regarded as positive when any one of the tests were abnormal but specificity would be reduced. Conversely, if a result were taken to be positive only when all tests were abnormal then specificity would be increased while reducing sensitivity. However, neither of these interpretations is optimal. A more sophisticated statistical technique is needed to maximise the information from each test. This has been attempted for the discrimination between benign and malignant masses using a combination of CA 125, ultrasound score and menopausal status [39]. Data were available prior to surgery on 101 women with benign and 42 with malignant pelvic masses. Ultrasound was scored 1 for each adverse feature present with a maximum of 3. Using stepwise logistic regression analysis a formula was derived which discriminated between benign and malignant lesions better than any other combination. The formula was simplified to the product of CA 125 and the score multiplied by 3 if the woman was post-menopausal. Using a 200 cut-off point, 85% of malignant lesions and only 3% of benign lesions were positive. Thus a positive result increased the chance of malignancy 28-fold and a negative result decreased it 6-fold.

Although statistical methods like this are impressive, they should be used with caution. The methods have the drawback that the derived formula will optimally fit the study data, but it is unlikely to fit a new series so well. This was found to be so for the above formula when it was applied to an independent series including 87 women with benign lesions and 37 malignant [55]. Using the same 200 cut-off point the proportion of malignant lesions yielding high scores was similar to the previous study (89%) but the fraction of benign lesions with positive results was increased to 13%.

Two groups have reported the use of discriminant analysis to combine information on a panel of several tumour markers including CA 125 measured consecutively: one used six markers [44] and the other used ten [46]. When the formula derived by the latter group was applied to the original series of 215 benign and 122 malignant ovarian tumours sensitivity was 84% and only 2.5% of those with benign lesions had positive results. However, when a fresh series was tested the proportions were 88% and 16%, respectively.

Targeting High Risk Populations

The positive predictive value of a screening test will be greater when it is applied to a population with higher than average prior risk of the disorder unless the test performs less well in them. There might therefore be an advantage in restricting ovarian cancer screening to such groups. Some high risk groups would be expected to include only a small proportion of the affected cases. While targeting them would limit the impact of screening they might provide a suitable population for evaluating the tests because of the smaller study size needed.

Older Women

The prior risk of ovarian cancer increases steeply between age 20 and 50 years, approximately doubling every 10 years; thereafter it levels off. About 95% of deaths from ovarian cancer occur after age 45 years and 85% after 55 years. Given that the incidence of benign ovarian disease decreases with age [73] there seems to be little value in screening before age 40 years and it may be preferable to begin at age 50 years in order to avoid screening many premenopausal women.

In general, it would be impractical to select women for screening on the basis of epidemiological features other than age but there is a substantial subset of older women who have low ovarian cancer risk. These are women who have had a hysterectomy (Table 6.5). Apart from their low prior risk they present problems when ultrasound is used for screening. The normal range of ovarian volume is very wide with an average intermediate between that of premenopausal and post-menopausal women. This is presumably because they form a mixed group some of whom would not yet have been naturally menopausal. The problem is compounded by a difficulty in distinguishing adhesions from ovarian tumours.

Table 6.5   Relative risk of ovarian cancer in women who have had a hysterectomy

Study	Number of ovaries	Hysterectomy rate		Relative risk (a)/(b)
		Ovarian cancer (a)	Control (b)	
New York [75]	NK	16% (24/150)	23% (68/300)	0.65
Rochester [5]	2	4% (4/114)	13% (53/411)	0.25
	1	0% (0/2)	51% (27/53)	0.00
Washington [49]	NK	1% (2/155)	28% (43/155)	0.04
Milan [30]	1 or 2	5% (8/161)	7% (40/561)	0.68
Boston [17]	1 or 2	7% (15/215)	9% (20/215)	0.73
Seattle [72]	1 or 2	26% (75/285)	22% (236/1089)	1.29
Stanford [74]	1 or 2	22% (41/188)	29% (154/539)	0.70
London [10]	2	4% (8/228)	14% (62/432)	0.22
	1	29% (2/7)	52% (10/19)	0.36

NK = not known

Symptomatic Cases

Women who are attending gynaecology clinics for various non-specific symptoms are at increased risk of ovarian cancer. Although the positive predictive value is likely to be high many would regard testing such women as clinical work-up rather than screening. Furthermore, the overall impact in the early diagnosis of ovarian cancer would be minimal. Nonetheless, intervention studies targeted on such a population will provide a better indication of sensitivity than obtained from observational studies carried out prior to surgery in woman with an ovarian mass.

Family History

A family history of ovarian cancer is associated with increased risk of the disease. There are believed to be three kinds of high risk pedigrees: site-specific familial ovarian cancer, breast–ovary families with a preponderance of these two cancer types and Lynch Syndrome II families in which there are cases of colon and endometrial as well as ovarian cancer. In a segregation analysis of 462 British pedigrees, the best fitting model was a rare autosomal dominant gene with 75%–79% penetrance [35]. This gene would account for the majority of ovarian cancer cases occurring at young ages. Consequently, women with a first degree relative diagnosed with ovarian cancer at a relatively young age, say under 55 years, constitute a high risk group. A gene on the long arm of chromosome 17 is now thought to be responsible for the breast–ovary families.

Despite the high risks involved, only a small proportion of ovarian cancers will occur in women with a significant family history or who are known to be gene carriers. Hence the identification of such women for screening would have little overall impact on ovarian cancer. Nonetheless they are a group motivated to be screened and because of the high incidence will generate more readily than the general population sufficient cancers to judge the sensitivity of a screening test. They are not a suitable group on which to carry out randomised trials since it is likely that assignment to a control arm would be unacceptable.

Intervention Studies

Several screening studies have now been undertaken in which the results have been used to judge whether or not to carry out abdominal surgery. Most have been demonstration projects to examine the feasibility of screening, many of them using a protocol expected to improve performance over that seen in the observational studies. None have attempted to address the central issue of whether screening reduces mortality although two pilot randomised trials have been described.

General Population

Five centres have reported the results of screening women selected only on the basis of their age and menopausal status.

King's College Hospital, London

A total of 5479 volunteers mostly aged 45 years or more were recruited in response to wide media publicity [13]. All had at least one transabdominal ultrasound screen; 90% had two routine repeat screens and 77% had three, at an average interval of about 18 months. If increased ovarian volume or abnormal morphology were found the examination was repeated 3–8 weeks later. Over the three screens an average of 2.3% were referred to a surgeon and five women were found to have primary ovarian cancer (all Stage I including one bilateral cancer) giving a positive predictive value of 1 in 67. Ovarian cancer was diagnosed in four additional women but this was found to be metastatic disease (two bilateral) from the breast or colon. Including all ovarian malignancies the positive predictive value was 1 in 37. One woman with negative ultrasound results presented clinically with ovarian cancer two years after the third ultrasound screening examination. Although the overall sensitivity appears to be high it should be noted that four of the nine screen-detected cancers were not found until the second round of screening.

Lexington, Kentucky

Annual transvaginal ultrasound was used to screen 1300 postmenopausal asymptomatic women [69]. Those with an ovarian volume exceeding $8 \, cm^3$ or with abnormal morphology were regarded as abnormal and investigated further. If the abnormality persisted after 4 weeks laparotomy was recommended. Thirty-three women (2.5%) had abnormal scans and 27 went on to have surgery. As a result two Stage I primary ovarian cancers were diagnosed (positive predictive value 1 in 14) and a third case was a metastasis from a hitherto undiagnosed cancer of the colon. One of the primary cancers was only detected on the third annual screen; it is not stated in publications from the group how many rounds of screening have been carried out. Apart from this case no false negative results have been reported.

In the initial phase of the study premenopausal women were also included [70]. The protocol was similar to that of the postmenopausal women except that a larger cut-off volume was used (18 cm³) and in those with enlargement but normal morphology the scan was repeated one week after the next menstrual period. Of the 39 (9.2%) who had abnormal scans, only 16 (3.8%) were persistently so. Laparotomy was performed on 13 and no malignancies were found.

Royal London Hospital

Postmenopausal women aged 45 years or older were recruited systematically from workforce and general practitioner lists as well as including self-selected individuals coming forward in response to press coverage of the project [38, 40]. The protocol was to perform a baseline CA 125 determination. Those with levels exceeding 30 U/ml were offered an ultrasound examination which assessed size and morphology. However, this was not a simple sequential design as CA 125 tests were repeated quarterly in women with a negative scan result and equivocal scans were repeated every 4–6 weeks.

In total 22 000 women were screened and 340 (1.5%) had raised baseline CA 125 levels. Twelve were subsequently found to have ovarian cancer, a positive predictive value of 1 in 28. The effect of sequential screening with ultrasound was to improve substantially the positive predictive value to 1 in 4 with only 41 women having laparotomy of whom 11 had ovarian cancer (the remaining woman had refused ultrasound). Seven further cases of ovarian cancer had surfaced as false-negative CA 125 results after two years of follow-up. Thus sensitivity was not high, especially for early disease. Three Stage I tumours were diagnosed at laparotomy compared with five presenting at follow-up (all had CA 125 under 15 U/ml). Moreover, the average lead time was unlikely to have been great.

Stockholm, Sweden

Women aged 40 years or older were selected from a population register to be offered screening with CA 125 [22]. If the result was positive the test was repeated quarterly and ultrasound with physical examination was performed biannually. In order to avoid biased interpretation of examinations a control group with normal CA 125 was also followed-up with the same regimen and the clinicians were blinded as to the levels.

A total of 5550 women were tested and 175 (3.2%) had elevated levels using 35 U/ml as cut-off in the initial phase and 30 U/ml thereafter. Six were found to have ovarian cancer, a positive predictive value for CA 125 of 1 in 29. However, the sequential regime was effective since in order to diagnose the six malignancies only 16 laparotomies were performed: an overall positive predictive value of 1 in 3. Retrospective analysis of the CA 125 results was performed to examine a policy of restricting screening to women age 50 years or more and regarding CA 125 as positive if the level exceeded 95 U/ml or was initially over 30 U/ml but doubled after repeat testing. Just 21 women would have been positive and all six ovarian cancers would have been detected with a positive predictive value of 1 in 4. Record linkage with cancer registry and in-patient files revealed six further cases of ovarian cancer in women with initially normal CA 125 levels. Hence sensitivity was not very high.

Zagreb, Croatia

A total of 743 postmenopausal asymptomatic women were screened using transvaginal ultrasound incorporating colour Doppler [47]. Either ovarian enlargement (exceeding 5 cm) or an ovarian mass with a low resistance index (under 0.4) on two separate occasions was used to identify women for surgery. Four malignant ovarian tumours were found; three were Stage I and one Stage III. There is no more detailed information concerning performance.

Gynaecology Outpatients

Lund, Sweden

Two series of women aged 40 years or more were offered routine transabdominal ultrasound when attending gynaecological outpatients clinics [2, 4]. A total of 1596 women attended largely because of symptoms, sometimes non-specific, and epidemiological risk factors. Those with enlarged ovaries (exceeding 2 cm) or abnormal morphology had a repeat scan 2–6 weeks later. Following a positive ultrasound result 97 (6%) had surgery which revealed ovarian cancer in 10, a positive predictive value of 1 in 10. Formal follow-up of women with negative ultrasound examinations was not undertaken but no further ovarian cancers were known to the authors between the study and the time of publication despite the hospital being the gynaecological referral centre for the area.

Other Series

Transvaginal ultrasound was used to screen 212 postmenopausal women in Gottingen, Germany [54]. Twenty-seven (13%) had an abnormality and two ovarian cancers were detected, a positive predictive value of 1 in 13. In Trieste, Italy, ultrasound was used on 500 women aged 45 years or more attending a clinic for cervical screening [51]. Eleven (2%) had an abnormality, six had surgery and no abnormalities were found.

Family History

King's College Hospital, London

Women age 25 years or older with at least one second degree relative or closer with ovarian cancer were offered an ultrasound screen [12]. A total of 1601 eligible women were recruited as a result of press publicity. Transvaginal sonography was used to identify abnormal morphology which persisted after a repeat scan 3–8 weeks later. Volume by itself was not a criterion for abnormality but if the volume was reduced by 63% or more at the repeat scan the result was regarded as negative despite persistent morphological change.

Overall 61 women (3.8%) had positive screening results and six primary ovarian cancers were detected (positive predictive value 1 in 10). Five of the tumours were at Stage I and one at Stage III. Over half the women were screened more than once but the published results do not make it clear at which round the cancers were detected. Women were followed-up by letter or telephone and three ovarian cancers had surfaced between 2 and 3½ years since the last scan.

Retrospective analysis of Doppler ultrasound results and morphology scores for women with abnormal scans suggested that a substantial improvement in positive predictive value is possible albeit at the cost of reduced sensitivity.

Yale, Connecticut

Women aged 35 years or over who have a first degree relative with ovarian cancer are being recruited [62]. The protocol is intense so that participants are seen every 3 months. At the first visit and every 6 months thereafter screening is by physical examination and a panel of tumour markers including CA 125. The next visit at 3 months and every 6 months thereafter is for a transvaginal ultrasound examination to determine morphology and vascularity by colour Doppler. If the level of any one marker is elevated the woman is tested again after one month. A further increase in the level by a given amount is regarded as a positive result.

So far only the results of the first 84 participants have been reported [63]. Three women (4%) have undergone laparotomy but only one was principally because of suspicion of ovarian cancer. No malignancies were present.

Los Angeles

A widespread publicity campaign has been used to recruit women age 35 years or more to a family cancer screening programme [41]. Eligibility is dependent on having at least one first degree relative with breast, colon or gynaecological cancer or a second degree relative with ovarian cancer. Transvaginal ultrasound is used to determine ovarian volume, morphology and blood flow. Five tumour markers are also used including CA 125. If an abnormal screening result is found the screen is repeated 6 months later.

A total of 597 asymptomatic women have been screened so far. One or more tests yielded an abnormal result in 115 women (19%) and 19 (3%) subsequently underwent oophorectomy. Only one of the women operated on was found to have ovarian cancer (Stage I).

Pilot Randomised Trials

Two trials – in Copenhagen and Reading, UK – have been in progress for some time but only preliminary details are so far available.

In Copenhagen women aged 45–64 years are recruited from population registers to be offered entry to the trial. Of 1557 eligible women, 64% expressed a willingness to join the study and 950 have been randomised to two equal sized study and control arms (A. Tabor, personal communication). Those in the study arm receive transvaginal ultrasound and a dual marker blood test (CA 125 and Tetranectin).

In Reading, women aged 50–61 years attending a breast screening centre for routine mammography are recruited to the trial. Among the first 1160 women invited 1002 (86%) agreed to randomisation between equal study and control arms [18]. Those in the study arm have an ultrasound scan. Initially both transvaginal and transabdominal scanning was used but practical problems were encountered with the latter. Transabdominal scanning requires a full bladder so that women could not usually be scanned on the same day as the mammography. Since the transvaginal method appeared to be acceptable to most women this alone was eventually adopted.

A European Community Concerted Action has now been formed to take the pilot studies a stage further. Four centres in addition to Copenhagen and Reading are to follow a common protocol using ultrasound alone. Women aged 55–64 years will be randomised to three arms: two screening arms of 20 000 each and 40 000 controls. After the baseline ultrasound those in the screening arms will be recalled either every 1½ or 3 years. Women with abnormal scan results will then have a Doppler ultrasound examination. The study is designed so that after 4 years' follow-up there will be enough power to detect an improvement in surrogate measures of screening efficacy such as the interval cancer rate. If these results are encouraging the aim would be to extend the pilot study into a full trial with mortality as the end-point.

Conclusions

Of the screening modalities currently available ultrasound appears to be the most sensitive although not sufficiently so for it to be used alone. A high positive predictive value is essential for ovarian cancer and a combination of different tests will be needed to achieve this together with targeting screening on those with the highest risk. Unbiased estimates of sensitivity and specificity cannot be obtained from the observational studies of women tested prior to surgery. Estimates derived from the intervention studies are not biased but the relatively small numbers of affected individuals and the unsystematic follow-up limits their value. The randomised trials of ultrasound should eventually provide reliable estimates. For these trials to be extended to full investigations of efficacy with mortality as the end-point the interim results would need to demonstrate that the positive predictive value is acceptable while maintaining a reasonable sensitivity. The results of the intervention studies reported so far do not provide encouragement that this can be achieved.

References

1. Anderson MC (1990) Malignant potential of benign ovarian cysts: the case "for". In: Sharp F, Mason WP, Leake RE (eds) Ovarian cancer. Chapman and Hall Medical, London, pp 187–190.
2. Andolf E, Jörgensen C, Astedt B (1990) Ultrasound examination for detection of ovarian carcinoma in risk groups. Obstet Gynecol 75:106–109.
3. Andolf E, Jörgensen C, Svalenius E et al. (1987) Ultrasound measurement of the ovarian volume. Acta Obstet Gynaecol Scand 66:387–389.
4. Andolf E, Svalenius E, Astedt B (1986) Ultrasonography for early detection of ovarian carcinoma. Br J Obstet Gynaecol 93:1286–1289.
5. Annegers JF, Strom H, Decker DG et al. (1979) Ovarian cancer. Incidence and case-control study. Cancer 43:723–729.
6. Ayalon D, Graif M, Hetman-Peri M et al. (1988) Diagnosis of a small ovarian tumor (androgen secreting) by magnetic resonance: A new noninvasive procedure. Am J Obstet Gynecol 159:903–905.
7. Bast RC, Klug TL, St John E et al. (1983) A radioimmunoassay using a monoclonal antibody to monitor the course of epithelial cancer. N Engl J Med 309:883–887.
8. Bast RC, Knauf S, Epenetos A et al. (1991) Coordinate elevation of serum markers in ovarian cancer but not in benign disease. Cancer 68:1758–1763.
9. Benaceraff BR, Finkler NJ, Wojciechowski C et al. (1990) Sonographic accuracy in the diagnosis of ovarian masses. J Reprod Med 5:491–495.
10. Booth M, Beral V, Smith P (1989) Risk factors for ovarian cancer: a case-control study. Br J Cancer 60:592–598.
11. Bourne T, Campbell S, Steer C et al. (1989) Transvaginal colour flow imaging: a possible new screening technique for ovarian cancer. Br Med J 299:1367–1370.
12. Bourne TH, Campbell S, Reynolds KM et al. (1993) Screening for early familial ovarian cancer with transvaginal ultrasonography and colour blood flow imaging. Br Med J 306:1025–1029.
13. Campbell S, Bhan V, Royston P et al. (1989) Transabdominal ultrasound screening for early ovarian cancer. Br Med J 299:1363–1367.
14. Campbell S, Collins WP, Royston P et al. (1990) Developments in ultrasound screening for early ovarian cancer. In: Sharp F, Mason WP, Leake RE (eds) Ovarian cancer. Chapman and Hall Medical, London, pp 217–227.
15. Chamberlain G, Brown JC (eds) (1978) Gynaecological laparoscopy. The report of the Working Party of the Confidential Enquiry in Gynaecological Laparoscopy. Royal College of Obstetricians and Gynaecologists, London.
16. Cole LA, Nam J-H, Chambers JT et al. (1990) Urinary gonadotropin fragment, a new tumor marker. Gynecol Oncol 36:391–394.
17. Cranmer DW, Hutchinson GB, Welch WR et al. (1983) Determinants of ovarian cancer risk. I. Reproductive experiences and family history. J Natl Cancer Inst 71:711–716.
18. Cuckle H, Wald N. (1991) Screening for ovarian cancer. In: Miller AB, Chamberlain J, Day NE, Hakama M, Prorok PC (eds) Cancer screening. Cambridge University Press, Cambridge, pp 228–239.
19. Cuckle HS, Wald NJ, Thompson SG (1987) Estimating a woman's risk of having a pregnancy associated with Down's syndrome using her age and serum alpha-feto-protein level. Br J Obstet and Gynaecol 94:387–402.
20. Devine PL, McGuckin MA, Ward BG (1992) Circulating mucins as tumor markers in

ovarian cancer (Review). Anticancer Res 12:709–718.

21. Diernaes E, Rasmussen J, Soerensen T et al. (1987) Ovarian cysts: management by puncture? Lancet i:1084.

22. Einhorn N, Sjövall K, Knapp RC et al. (1992) Prospective evaluation of serum CA 125 levels for early detection of ovarian cancer. Obstet Gynecol 80:14–18.

23. Ferdeghini M, Gadducci A, Prontera C et al. (1992) Combined evaluation of serum CA 125 and CAM 29 in patients with epithelial ovarian cancer. Tumor Biol 13:287–293.

24. Finkler NJ, Benacerraf B, Lavin PT et al. (1988) Comparison of serum CA 125, clinical impression, and ultrasound in the preoperative evaluation of ovarian masses. Obstet Gynecol 72:659–64.

25. Fisken J, Roulston JE, Sturgeon C et al. (1993) The value of the human milk fat globule membrane antigen $HMFG_2$ in epithelial ovarian cancer monitoring: comparison with CA 125. Br J Cancer 67:1065–1070.

26. Fleisher AC, Rogers WH, Rao BK et al. (1991) Transvaginal color Doppler sonography of ovarian masses with pathological correlation. Ultrasound Obstet Gynecol 1:275–278.

27. Folke Pettersen (ed) (1988) Annual Report on the results of treatment in Gynaecological cancer. 20th Vol. International Federation of Gynaecology and Obstetrics.

28. Folkman J, Watson K, Ingber D et al. (1989) Introduction of angiogenesis during the transition from hyperplasia to neoplasia. Nature 339:58–61

29. Fox H. (1990) Malignant potential of benign ovarian cysts: the case "against". In: Sharp F, Mason WP, Leake RE (eds) Ovarian cancer. Chapman and Hall Medical, London, pp 185–186.

30. Franceschi S, La Vecchia C, Helmrich SP et al. (1982) Risk factors for epithelial ovarian cancer in Italy. Am J Epidemiol 115:714–719.

31. Gadducci A, Ferdeghini M, Ceccarini T et al. (1989) The serum concentrations of TAG-72 antigen measured with CA 72-4 IRMA in patients with ovarian carcinoma. Preliminary data. J Nuclear Med Allied Sci 33:32–36.

32. Goswamy RK, Campbell S, Royston JP (1988) Ovarian size in postmenopausal women. Br J Obstet Gynaecol 95:795–801.

33. Hata K, Hata T, Senoh D et al. (1989) Doppler ultrasound assessment of tumour vascularity in gynecologic disorders. J Ultrasound Med 8:299–308.

34. Hata K, Hata T, Manabe A et al. (1992) A critical evaluation of transvaginal Doppler studies, transvaginal sonography, magnetic resonance imaging, and CA 125 in detecting ovarian cancer. Obstet Gynecol 80:922–926.

35. Houlston RS, Collins A, Slack J et al. (1991) Genetic epidemiology of ovarian cancer: segregation analysis. Ann Hum Genet 55:291–299.

36. Hricak H, Lacey C, Schriock E et al. (1985) Gynecologic masses: value of magnetic resonance imaging. Am J Obstet Gynecol 153:31–37.

37. Jacobs I, Bast RC (1989) The CA 125 tumour-associated antigen: a review of the literature. Hum Reprod 4:1–12.

38. Jacobs I, Davies AP, Bridges J et al. (1993) Prevalence screening for ovarian cancer in postmenopausal women by CA 125 measurement and ultrasonography. Br Med J 306:1030–1034.

39. Jacobs I, Oram D, Fairbanks J et al. (1990) A risk of malignancy index incorporating CA 125, ultrasound and menopausal status for the accurate preoperative diagnosis of ovarian cancer. Br J Obstet Gynaecol 97:922–929

40. Jacobs IJ, Stabile I, Bridges J et al. (1988) Multimodal approach to screening for ovarian cancer. Lancet i:268–271.

41. Karlan BY, Raffel LJ, Crvenkovic G et al. (1993) A multidisciplinary approach to the early detection of ovarian carcinoma: rationale, protocol design, and early results. Am J Obstet Gynecol 169:494–501.
42. Kawai M, Kano R, Kikkawa F et al. (1992) Transvaginal Doppler ultrasound with color flow imaging in the diagnosis of ovarian cancer. Obstet Gynecol 79:163–167.
43. Kobayashi H, Ohi H, Fujii R et al. (1993) Characterisation and clinical usefulness of CA130 antigen recognised by monoclonal antibodies, 130-22 and 145-9, in ovarian cancer. Br J Cancer 67:237–243.
44. Kobayashi H, Sumimoto K, Terao T et al. (1992) Field trial for the early detection of patients with ovarian cancer – discrimination of ovarian cancer patients by the statistical analysis using Mahalanobis' generalized distance. (In Japanese) Acta Obstet Gynaecol Japonica 44:174–180.
45. Kobayashi H, Tamura M, Satoh T et al. (1993) Clinical evaluation of new cancer-associated antigen CA125 II in epithelial ovarian cancers: comparison with CA125. Clin Biochem 26:213–219.
46. Kobayashi S, Murae M, Kimura E (1993) Development and clinical research of computer aided multivariate pattern analysis system (CAMPAS) OV-1 for diagnosis of ovarian carcinoma. (In Japanese) Acta Obstet Gynaecol Japonica 45:241–248.
47. Kurjak A, Schulman H, Sosic A et al. (1992) Transvaginal ultrasound, color flow, and Doppler waveform of the postmenopausal adnexal mass. Obstet Gynecol 80:917–921.
48. Kurjak A, Zalud I, Alfirevic Z et al. (1990) The assessment of abnormal pelvic blood flow by transvaginal color and pulsed Doppler. Ultrasound Med Biol 16:437–442
49. McGowan L, Parent L, Lednar W et al. (1979) The woman at risk for developing ovarian cancer. Gynecol Oncol 7:325–44
50. Meire HB, Farrant P, Guha T (1978) Distinction of benign from malignant ovarian cysts by ultrasound. Br J Obstet Gynaecol 85:893–899.
51. Millo R, Facca MC, Alberico S (1989) Sonographic evaluation of ovarian volume in postmenopausal women: a screening test for ovarian cancer? Clin Exp Obstet Gynecol 2-3:72–78.
52. Molina R, Ojeda B, Filella X et al. (1992) A prospective study of tumor markers CA 125 and CA 19.9 in patients with epithelial ovarian carcinomas. Tumor Biol 13:278–286.
53. Negishi Y, Iwabuchi H, Sakunaga H et al. (1993) Serum and tissue measurements of CA72-4 in ovarian cancer patients. Gynecol Oncol 48:148–154.
54. Osmers R, Völksen M, Rath W et al. (1989) Die Vaginalsonographie: eine Screening-methode zur Früherkennung von Ovarialtumoren und Endometriumkarzinomen? Arch Gynecol Obstet 245:602–606.
55. Prys Davies A, Jacobs I, Wollas R et al. (1993) The adnexal mass: benign or malignant? Evaluation of a risk of malignancy index. Br J Obstet and Gynaecol 100:927–931.
56. Rodriguez MH, Platt LD, Medearis AL et al. (1988) The use of transvaginal sonography for evaluation of postmenopausal ovarian size and morphology. Am J Obstet Gynecol 159:810–814.
57. Rulin MC, Preston AL (1987) Adnexal masses in postmenopausal women. Obstet Gynecol 70:578–581.
58. Sanders RC, McNeil BJ, Finberg HJ et al. (1983) A prospective study of computer tomography and ultrasound in the detection and staging of pelvic masses. Radiology 146:439–442.
59. Sassone AM, Timor-Tritsch IE, Artner A et al. (1991) Transvaginal sonographic characterization of ovarian disease: evaluation of a new scoring system to predict ovarian malignancy. Obstet Gynecol 78:70–76.

60. Scambia G, Panici PB, Perrone L et al. (1990) Serum levels of tumour associated glycoprotein (TAG 72) in patients with gynaecological malignancies. Br J Cancer 62:147–151.

61. Schwartz PE, Chambers SK, Chambers JT et al. (1987) Circulating tumor markers in the monitoring of gynecologic malignancies. Cancer 60:353–361.

62. Schwartz PE, Chambers JT, Taylor KJ et al. (1991) Early detection of ovarian cancer: background, rationale, and structure of the Yale Early Detection Program. Yale J Biol Med 64:557–571

63. Schwartz PE, Chambers JT, Taylor KJ et al. (1991) Early detection of ovarian cancer: preliminary results of the Yale Early Detection Program. Yale J Biol Med 64:573–582.

64. Shepherd JH, Granowska M, Britton KE et al. (1987) Tumour-associated monoclonal antibodies for the diagnosis and assessment of ovarian cancer. Br J Obstet Gynaecol 94:160–167.

65. Smith LH, Oi RH (1984) Detection of malignant ovarian neoplasms: a review of the literature. Obstet Gynecol Surv 39:313–360.

66. Suzuki M, Sekiguchi I, Tamada T (1990) Clinical evaluation of tumor-associated mucin-type glycoprotein CA 54/61 in ovarian cancers: comparison with CA 125. Obstet Gynecol 76:422–427.

67. Takeuchi H, Kawamata C, Sugie T et al. (1978) Grey scale ultrasonic diagnosis of ovarian carcinoma. Excerpta Medica International Congress Series 436:113–121.

68. Timor-Tritsch IE, Lerner JP, Monteagudo A et al. (1993) Transvaginal ultrasonographic characterization of ovarian masses by means of color flow-directed Doppler measurements and a morphologic scoring system. Am J Obstet Gynecol 168:909–913.

69. van Nagell JR, DePriest PD, Puls LE et al. (1991) Ovarian cancer screening in asymptomatic postmenopausal women by transvaginal sonography. Cancer 68:458–462.

70. van Nagell JR, Higgins RV, Donaldson ES et al. (1990) Transvaginal sonography as a screening method for ovarian cancer: a report of the first 1000 cases screened. Cancer 65:573–577.

71. Weiner Z, Thaler I, Beck D et al. (1992) Differentiating malignant from benign ovarian tumors with transvaginal color flow imaging. Obstet Gynecol 79:159–162.

72. Weiss NS, Harlow BL (1986) Why does hysterectomy without bilateral oophorectomy influence the subsequent incidence of ovarian cancer? Am J Epidemiol 124:856–858.

73. Westhoff CL, Beral V (1984) Patterns of ovarian cyst hospital discharge rates in England and Wales, 1962–79. Br Med J 289:1348–1349.

74. Wu ML, Whittemore AS, Paffenbarger RS et al. (1988) Personal and environmental characteristics related to epithelial ovarian cancer. Am J Epidemiol 128:1216–1227.

75. Wynder EL, Dodo H, Barber HRG (1969) Epidemiology of cancer of the ovary. Cancer 23:352–370.

76. Xu F-J, Ramakrishnan S, Daly L et al. (1991) Increased serum levels of macrophage colony-stimulating factor in ovarian cancer. Am J Obstet Gynecol 165:1356–1362.

77. Yemeda KA, Kenemans P, Wobbes T et al. (1991) Carcinoma-associated mucin serum markers CA M26 and CA M29: Efficacy in detecting and monitoring patients with cancer of the breast, colon, ovary, endometrium and cervix. Int J Cancer 47:170–179.

78. Zurawski VR, Orjaseter H, Andersen A, Jellum E (1988) Elevated serum CA 125 levels prior to diagnosis of ovarian neoplasia: relevance for early detection of ovarian cancer. Int J Cancer 42:677–680.

79. Zurawski VR, Sjovall K, Schoenfeld DA et al. (1990) Prospective evaluation of serum CA 125 levels in a normal population, phase I: the specificities of single and serial determinations in testing for ovarian cancer. Gynecol Oncol 36:299–305.

7 – Screening for Prostate Cancer

Jocelyn Chamberlain and Jane Melia

Prostate cancer is a large and increasing problem in the developed world. With around 11 000 new cases and 8 000 deaths each year in England and Wales it is the fourth commonest cancer in men (after lung, skin and large bowel) and the second commonest cause of cancer death (after lung cancer). It is primarily a disease of the elderly, with 73% of new cases, and 80% of prostate cancer deaths occurring in men over the age of 70 years.

Time Trends and International Differences in Incidence

The frequency of prostate cancer has been increasing in the UK, as in other developed countries. In England and Wales the registration rate of new cases in 1987 was 44.2 per 100 000 males, an increase of 14% over the 1979 rate [36]. The increase occurred in all age-groups over 50 years but was most marked among men over 75 years. Mortality has also been increasing, the 1992 crude death rate of 30.3 per 100 000 males being 13% higher than that ten years earlier in 1983 [37]. There may be spurious explanations for part of these trends, such as increasingly accurate diagnosis of the cause of death in elderly men and increasing completeness of ascertainment of new cases by cancer registries. Nevertheless there can be little doubt that part, at least, of the increase is real, and these trends are also seen in the rest of the world [12].

There are very interesting differences in the incidence of prostate cancer in different countries. In an international comparison of different cancer registries [35], incidence rates for the period 1978–1982, age-adjusted to a World Standard population to make them comparable, were highest in US Blacks (91.2 per 100 000 in the Atlanta Cancer Registry) and lowest in the Far East (1.8 per 100 000 in China, and 5.1 per 100 000 in Japan). Table 7.1 shows some of the cancer registries with incidence rates between these two extremes. The fact that Japanese who have migrated to Hawaii have intermediate rates between those of Japan and the US has led to the hypothesis that environmental and cultural factors contribute to the aetiology of prostate cancer, playing a larger role than genetic factors.

The rising trend in prostate cancer incidence has been more marked than the trend in mortality, particularly in the USA, where prostate cancer is now even more frequent than lung cancer in men. The increasing gap between incidence and mortality is not thought to be due to greater successes of treatment since the methods used for treatment have not changed much over the past few decades. In recent years part of the rise in incidence is attributable to screening which is now widely prescribed in the US, but diverging trends of incidence and mortality pre-dated the introduction of screening by several years. Diagnosis of incidental prostate cancer following surgery for benign prostatic disease is probably a major contributor to the difference. Transurethral prostatectomy (TURP) is increasingly used to relieve urinary obstruction in men with benign prostatic hypertrophy (BPH), and it is common practice for the excised glandular tissue to be examined histologically, leading to increased detection of localised carcinoma. This "case-finding" of incidental prostate cancer in men with BPH is in many ways analogous to screening.

Table 7.1 Age-standardised incidence rates of prostate cancer in the period 1978–82 [35]

Country (cancer registry)	New registrations of prostate cancer per 100 000 men
US Blacks (Atlanta)	91.2
Canada (Saskatchewan)	57.6
US Whites (Atlanta)	53.2
Switzerland (Basel)	50
Sweden	45.9
Australia (NSW)	33.8
US Japanese (Hawaii)	31.2
UK (SE Scotland)	26.5
Italy (Varese)	20.3
UK (West Midlands)	18.9
Poland (Cracow)	13.8
India (Bombay)	8.2
Japan (Osaka)	5.1
China (Shanghai)	1.8

Potosky et al. [39] examined the association between prostate cancer incidence in four cancer registries contributing to the US National Cancer Institute Surveillance Epidemiology and End-Results Program (SEER), and the rate of transurethral pros-tatectomy in the same populations, derived from the National Hospital Discharge Survey and Veterans Administration hospital discharge summaries. Over a 14-year period from 1973 to 1986 there was a 30% increase in total prostate cancer registra-tion rates, and a 60% increase in localised prostate cancer registration rates. Using regression analysis, it was found that 88% of the incidence trend could be explained by the increase in TURP discharge rates. Moreover it was possible to estimate the proportion of men undergoing TURP who were discharged with a diagnosis of prostate cancer, and by subtracting these from the total incidence the trend in incidence *not* associated with TURP could be estimated and was found to be virtually flat. However, although concluding that increasing use of TURP is the main reason for increasing incidence in the US up to 1986, the authors point out that mortality has also risen, particularly in non-whites, and this suggests that the risk of prostate cancer has also been increasing. No conclusion could be drawn from this study about the effect of identifying and removing incidental carcinomas, whose natural history is uncertain, on later mortality.

Aetiology

A number of factors have been explored in attempts to identify risk factors for prostatic cancer and hence to find methods of primary prevention and/or target populations for screening. As already shown migrant studies indicate that environmental factors are likely to play a greater role than genetic susceptibility. Nevertheless a family history of prostate cancer confers increased risk, one study [48] having found a relative risk of 2.0 (95% CI 1.2–2.3) if one first degree relative is affected rising to 8.8 (95% CI 2.8–28.1) if both first and second degree relatives are affected. Moreover, as with other cancers with an inherited component, the age of onset of familial cases is lower than that of sporadic cases. It has been estimated that inherited cases comprise 43% of prostate cancers diagnosed under the age of 55 falling to 9% of those diagnosed over the age of 80 years [5]. It can be anticipated that relevant genetic mutations will be identified within the next few years.

The great majority of prostate cancers are sporadic and the predisposing causes are largely obscure. The principal environmental and social factors that have been investigated are occupation, diet, sexual habits and sexually transmitted infections [4]. Among occupations, workers with cadmium and other heavy metals are at increased risk, and some, but not all, studies have indicated that farmers may have increased risk. Recently an increased risk has been identified in men occupationally exposed to a number of radionuclides [43].

Of dietary factors, fat intake has been associated with prostate cancer, both in international correlations and in a majority of case-control studies. Beta-carotene consumption seems to be protective, as for other epithelial tumours, but with less effect in men aged over 75 years. Of sexual factors, age at first intercourse, frequency of intercourse, number of sexual partners and history of sexually transmitted disease have all been associated with some elevation of risk, but these findings are not consistent across all studies. Similarly some, but not all studies have found a positive association between vasectomy and subsequent prostate cancer risk.

Endogenous hormones influence the normal prostate, and hormonal therapy is, at least initially, effective in treatment of metastatic prostate cancer. The possible aetiological role of a large number of hormones, including testosterone, dihydrotestosterone, prolactin, follicle stimulating hormone, oestradiol, oestrone, luteinising hormone and sex hormone binding globulin, has been extensively researched in numerous studies comparing men with prostate cancer with age-matched controls. The results have been conflicting or inconclusive [4]. Various reasons may account for this, including the fact that, in general, serum levels of total hormone have been measured rather than free (unbound) hormone; the hormone levels may not have been measured in the same way, e.g. at the same time of day, in cases and controls; the levels in cases may have been influenced by the disease itself; and some of the smaller studies lacked statistical power. In spite of this tantalising failure to identify with certainty the relationship between hormone levels and prostate cancer there is a widespread belief that hormone manipulation could provide a means of primary prevention. Indeed one chemoprevention trial is already starting, using finasteride which blocks the activity of 5-alpha-reductase, an enzyme which is needed to convert testosterone into dihydrotestosterone [21].

A history of benign prostatic hypertrophy has also been investigated as a potential risk factor. However, the association between the two conditions, as already seen, is in large part due to diagnostic bias in that surgery for BPH leads to diagnosis of otherwise silent prostate cancer. BPH occurs in the central zone of the prostate whereas carcinoma arises in the peripheral zone so progression of benign hypertrophy to neoplasia is unlikely. However, the two conditions may have similar as yet unidentified hormonal stimuli.

Staging

Using the TNM staging system, the following categories of prostate cancer are recognised:

T0   Incidental or latent cancers, usually asymptomatic (may also include carcinoma-in situ)
T1   Palpable unilobar nodule less than 2 cm in diameter
T2   Palpable unilobar nodule greater than 2 cm in diameter, or bilobar or multifocal nodules
T3   Palpable tumour with extraprostatic spread extending less than 5 cm
T4   Palpable tumour with greater than 5 cm extension to the bladder neck or pelvic side-wall
N+   Any size tumour with involved regional lymph nodes
M+   Any size tumour with distant metastatic disease

In North America the Whitmore Jewett system, with rubrics A to D, is more commonly used but is essentially similar. Stage A, equivalent to T0, is sometimes subdivided into A1 called "focal" (tumour present in not more than 5% of TURP histology chips) and A2 called "diffuse" (tumour present in more than 5% of chips) because it is believed that the latter group of larger volume tumours require more aggressive treatment. The inaccuracy of clinical staging is well demonstrated in one large French study [27] in which histological findings following radical prostatectomy resulted in upgrading 25% of clinical Stage T1 patients and 50% of clinical Stage T3. Only 2% were downstaged. It is now recognised that, not only clinical staging, but also morphological and imaging investigations are not very reliable in distinguishing different prognostic categories on which to base therapeutic decisions [40].

Few clinical series have reported their distribution of different stages at diagnosis in the totality of prostate cancers, most focusing only on subgroups receiving different forms of therapy. In a 1980 review of 100 consecutive patients presenting to a urology department in Edinburgh 23% were T0, 1% T1, 13% T2, 52% T3 and 11% T4 [10]. A US survey, over a 10-year period from 1973 to 1983 reported that 27% of patients presenting with symptoms were Stage A (T0), 28% Stage B (T1/T2) and 38% Stages C or D (T3/T4) (7% were unknown stage) [45]. When comparing percentage stage distributions in different studies it is important to remember that a high proportion of Stage A (T0) cases automatically lowers the percentage of other stages, even though the actual incidence rate of later stages may be no different in the populations reported in different series. Population-based stage-specific incidence rates have been reported from areas covered by the Surveillance, Epidemiology and End-Results (SEER) cancer registries in the USA [31]. Stage was classified as local, regional or distant. Among white males aged 50–79 years, during the period 1983–1987, there was an annual average increase of 5.9% in localised prostate cancer (accounting for two-thirds of the overall growth in incidence) and an increase of 10.6% in regional prostate cancer, but no increase in the incidence of metastatic disease. In 1987, the incidence rates of metastatic disease and of regional disease were similar at around 0.5 per 1000, whereas the incidence of localised disease was four times greater at about two per 1000. These US figures, as already seen, are influenced by the frequency of incidental prostate cancers diagnosed during surgery for benign prostatic hypertrophy, and probably to some extent also by screening which was already being implemented.

Survival

Overall, the 5-year survival of patients with prostate cancer diagnosed in England and Wales in 1981 was 43% [36]. As expected, survival varies with stage. An American series found that 5-year survival decreased from 89% for Stage A1 disease to 26% for Stage D2 [45]. In patients with metastases, although hormonal treatment usually leads to a temporary remission, the tumour soon becomes hormone resistant for reasons which are not understood, and case fatality is high, with a 5-year survival rate as low as 15% [19]. There is some evidence both from cancer registry data and from some clinical series that survival is also related to age, with poorer relative survival rates among men younger than 65 years at diagnosis and also in those aged over 75 years [55]. When examined by stage it is found that although younger men have better relative survival for localised disease than their older counterparts, their survival rates are worse for non-localised tumours. This may be due to late diagnosis because of failure to suspect the disease in younger men, or to a higher degree of malignancy within clinical stage at younger ages.

The influence of treatment on survival of earlier stages of the disease is controversial and, surprisingly, has not been sufficiently evaluated by randomised clinical trials of alternative therapies. The two principal local treatments which may be applied with curative intent to non-metastatic patients are radical prostatectomy or radical radiotherapy. Systemic treatment by hormonal manipulation (orchidectomy or administration of anti-androgens) is the treatment of first choice for metastatic disease. Five-year survival rates of 90% or more have been reported for patients with localised disease treated by radical prostatectomy, and for those treated by external beam radiotherapy [7, 22]. However, these results are not based on randomised trials and the different criteria of selection of patients for each treatment invalidates comparison between them.

Neither of these treatments are without serious side-effects, and concern about their appropriateness for localised prostate cancers led many clinicians to advocate a conservative "watch and wait" policy. Over a 7-year period George [19] followed 120 patients, free from metastases at time of diagnosis, with no anticancer therapy other than relief of urinary obstruction where necessary, and reported a 5-year actuarial survival rate of 80% excluding deaths from other causes. A number of other studies have reported similar findings, the most impressive of which is that by Johannson et al., in Sweden [24]. They followed-up a series of 223 patients from a defined population who had clinical Stage T0–T2, and Mo prostate cancer over a mean observation period of 123 months. A total of 76 patients (34%) experienced progression of disease but this was mainly localised and only 26 (12%) developed metastases. Nineteen (8.5%) died from prostate cancer, and 105 of other causes. In survival analyses, deaths from other causes were treated as censored events and proportional hazard analyses were performed to explore factors affecting case-fatality and disease progression. Age at diagnosis was not associated with either outcome, size of primary tumour was positively related to risk of disease progression but not to prostate cancer death, but histological grade was a strong determinant of both progression and death. A subgroup of 58 patients aged under 70 years and with Grade I or II tumours, who would have been eligible for radical prostatectomy under Swedish guidelines, were analysed separately and were found to have a greater risk of progression but not of prostate cancer death. The authors conclude that in the light of this evidence the high survival rates from uncontrolled studies of radical surgery or radiotherapy cannot be taken to be a favourable treatment effect. They report that a randomised controlled trial comparing radical prostatectomy with observation is in progress in Sweden and Finland, and another comparing irradiation with no initial treatment is underway in Denmark.

Natural History

From what is known from these studies of clinical prostate cancer it is apparent that there must be a wide range of growth rates in prostate cancer. This conclusion is reinforced when autopsy studies are also taken into account. It has been known for 60 years [41] that carcinoma of the prostate can be found in a proportion of men who die from unrelated causes. Numerous autopsy studies have confirmed this finding, and have also shown that the proportion increases with increasing age so that two-thirds or more of men aged over 65 years may have evidence of latent prostatic cancer [16].

The international variation in prostatic cancer has stimulated international comparisons of latent cancer at autopsy. One study [56] of the prevalence of prostate cancer at autopsy, using standardised methods, compared prostates from men aged over 50 years with no prior prostate surgery or diagnosis of prostate cancer, who died of unrelated conditions in New Orleans (178 blacks and 253 whites), in Colombia (182), in Hawaii (417 Japanese) and in Japan (576). The age-adjusted overall prevalence of latent prostate cancer was significantly higher in US blacks (36.9%), US Whites (34.6%) and Colombians (31.5%) than in Japanese in Japan (20.5%) but there was no significant difference between the rate in Hawaiian

Japanese (25.6%) and those in Japan. All cases of latent prostate cancer were classified histologically by two independent pathologists, into two types, latent infiltrative type and latent non-infiltrative type. There was no consistent relationship with race or with age in the prevalence of non-infiltrative type latent tumours, but infiltrative type tumours accounted for the entire differences in prevalence in the total sample. The infiltrative tumours were significantly larger than the non-infiltrative type in all races and their size increased with increasing age. Whitemore at al [54] used data from this and other autopsy studies together with cancer registration data to construct a natural history model which they conclude is consistent with the hypothesis that the volume of low-grade latent prostate cancer at any age determines the incidence rate of clinical cancer about 7 years later.

Determinants of Prognosis

A number of different diagnostic methods have been put forward in attempts to resolve the dilemma of which non-metastatic tumours require active treatment and which can be managed by surveillance. The patient's age and co-morbidity are clearly important indicators of his life-expectancy from which the probability of death from other causes before significant progression of the prostate cancer can be assessed.

Histopathological indicators of the likelihood of progression include tumour volume and histological grade. Assessment of tumour volume of incidental prostate cancer found in TURP specimens is based on the proportion of histology chips containing tumour. For preoperative assessment of tumour volume, transrectal ultrasound imaging may be used but, when compared with the cancer volume in subsequent radical prostatectomy specimens, has been shown to underestimate volume in a majority of tumours. Instead the degree to which each of six random-systematic ultrasound-guided biopsies is found to contain cancer indicates the extent of the tumour, as well as providing material for histological grading. Moreover, it is claimed that systematic biopsies do not lead to overdetection of very low volume clinically irrelevant prostate cancers [49].

Histological grade can be measured using classifications such as the Gleason score, in which scores up to 4 indicate well-differentiated tumours with low malignant potential, 5–7 intermediate, and 8–10 poor differentiation and high malignant potential; or the Mostofi system with just three grades: G1 well-differentiated, G2 moderately differentiated and G3 poorly differentiated. In a study of 80 untreated patients with non-metastatic prostate cancer, progression occurred in two out of five G3 tumours, in eight out of 32 G2 tumours, and in only one out of 43 G1 tumours [52]. Similarly Johannson et al. [24] found grade to be the only important determinant of risk of prostate cancer death.

Levels of prostate specific antigen (PSA) in serum increase with increasing tumour volume and are of accepted clinical value in predicting recurrence after treatment. Every 1 g of tumour (whether in the prostate or extracapsular) leads to an average elevation of PSA level of 3.5 ng/ml [47]. In a study of changes over time in PSA levels in a series of 43 patients with untreated prostate cancer this finding was used to derive doubling-times of tumour volume [44]. In six patients

(14%) with stable disease the PSA level did not increase, but in the remainder there was an exponential log-linear increase in PSA volume with time. Initial PSA values were lowest (median value 6.7 ng/ml) in the 17 patients with clinically confined cancer throughout the follow-up period, and their median doubling time was 69.3 months. For the 15 patients with T3, T4 or MO cancer, the median PSA level was 30.8 and median doubling-time 43 months. Three out of four patients who had distant metastases had doubling times of less than 12 months. The authors suggest that the initial PSA level, combined with the results of six random biopsies and the Gleason grade can confidently distinguish a tumour volume of less than 0.5 ml below which threshold active treatment can be withheld; and that such patients can be followed up by serial PSA measurements alone.

It can be expected that cytogenetic and molecular markers will be developed within the next few years to enable more accurate distinction of good prognosis from poor prognosis tumours and hence to tailor treatment policies more precisely [29].

Screening Tests for Prostate Cancer

There are three tests which have been used to screen for asymptomatic prostate cancer – digital rectal examination, serum prostate-specific antigen level, and transrectal ultrasound – each of which has been used both separately and in different combinations.

Digital Rectal Examination (DRE)

This classical technique for the diagnosis of prostate cancer (and incidentally rectal carcinoma) involves palpating the prostate gland to identify discrete nodular lesions or areas of induration and to assess the size of the gland. Only the posterior and lateral lobes of the gland can be adequately examined by digital rectal examination so that malignant lesions in the anterior and medial lobes will inevitably be missed. Although the majority of prostate cancers found by DRE are clinically localised, subsequent diagnostic work-up and histology of surgical specimens has been shown to result in reclassification to a more advanced stage in 50% [11] to 66% [50] of cases. Thus the proportion of cancers detectable by DRE at a curable stage is limited [42]. Detection of late-stage incurable cancer by screening confers no benefit, but rather lengthens the period of morbidity for the patient. Digital rectal examination used on its own also gives a substantial proportion of false positive results (i.e. abnormalities requiring further investigation). Its specificity is 94%–97%, and the positive predictive value of an abnormal DRE is 25%–39%.

Prostate Specific Antigen (PSA)

Prostate specific antigen is a protein found in healthy prostate epithelium and secreted into seminal fluid. Its expression is known to be controlled by androgens but its physiological function is unclear. Using PSA immunoassays it can be detected in serum and the serum level is increased in benign prostatic hypertrophy (BPH) and in primary and metastatic prostate cancer.

As a screening test it is simple and relatively cheap, requiring only a blood sample sent to a laboratory with a facility for conducting the assay. Unlike DRE and TRUS it is independent of the examiner's skill although of course quality control within the laboratory is essential. Being a quantitative measure its sensitivity and specificity can be altered by changing the cut-off level for distinguishing positive from negative. Catalona et al. [8] compared sensitivity and specificity for cut-off levels of 4.0 and 10 ng/ml in screening 1653 men aged over 50 years among whom 37 prostate cancers were found. All 37 cancers were found to have levels of 4 ng (100% sensitivity) but only 18 had levels of 10 µg or more (sensitivity 49%). Estimates of specificity were 96% and 99%, respectively. However, since those men with levels less than 4.0 ng/ml were not further investigated, it is possible that some cancers were not detected and that, for a cut-off level of 4 ng/ml, sensitivity was lower than 100%.

PSA values have been shown to increase with increasing age [23] so that different cut-off levels in screening men of different age-groups might be more appropriate. Part of this variability with age might be attributable to unrecognised benign prostatic hypertrophy since this too leads to elevation of PSA level. Armbruster, in a review of PSA [2] cited 10 studies of serum levels in patients with BPH in the largest of which over 20% of patients had levels of more than 4 ng/ml and 2%–3% levels greater than 10 ng/ml [26].

Carter et al. [6] have looked back at past serum PSA levels in men who subsequently developed prostate cancer, men who underwent surgery for benign prostatic hypertrophy and controls who, on examination, had no evidence of prostate disease. All of these men had been participants for at least 7 years in a longitudinal research study of ageing in which serum samples were obtained at 2-yearly intervals and stored. Among the cancer patients, 78% had had at least one PSA measurement greater than 4.0 ng/l, but so did 40% of subjects with BPH and 6.3% of controls. The availability of serial serum samples enabled Carter et al. to look not merely at a single reading above the chosen cut-off point, but at the rate of change over time. They found a gradient in the rate of change in PSA from a small increase, accounted for by increasing age, in the controls, to a faster rate in the BPH patients, faster still in the patients who developed localised prostate cancer, and greatest in the patients who subsequently developed metastatic prostate cancer. A cut-off criterion of an average rate of change of PSA greater than 0.75 ng/ml/year maintained the same 78% sensitivity but increased specificity to 90%.

The relevance of this finding to general population screening is uncertain, because it is based on a highly compliant group of volunteers who gave repeated serum samples every 2 years. Moreover the serum was tested retrospectively and thus the investigators did not have to confront the problem of what action to take on a single sample above a suspicious cut-off level. However, among men participating regularly in a screening programme, after the first screening round the rate of change in PSA measurement up to the chosen cut-off point could be calculated and might improve specificity. Moreover the ability of rate of change to predict who will develop metastatic disease may prove useful in deciding who needs radical treatment rather than observation. Similar nested case-control studies, based on serum banks, are currently underway in Finland and in the UK.

Transrectal Ultrasound (TRUS)

This test involves insertion of an ultrasound transducer into the rectum and scanning in both transverse and longitudinal directions. The anatomy of the gland can be visualised and its volume measured. TRUS identifies hypoechoic areas which are characteristic of carcinomas. In most studies it has been combined with digital rectal examination and/or PSA, although one Japanese study used it as a single modality in screening 6529 men, among whom 42 cancers were found at the expense of over 400 biopsies [53].

Because TRUS is capable of detecting some tumours which are impalpable, its use complements DRE, as has been shown in several studies in symptomatic patients, and volunteers [13]. In some series, it has been found to be more sensitive than DRE alone [28], in others less sensitive [51]. Probably the closest approximation to its use in screening asymptomatic populations comes from the American Cancer Society's National Cancer Detection Project [32]. Among 2425 volunteers aged 55–70 years, screened by TRUS and DRE, 57 cancers were found. TRUS detected 44 (sensitivity 77%) and DRE 33 (sensitivity 58%). But the specificity of TRUS was low at 0.89 and positive predictive value only 15%.

Because of its complexity, expense and requirement for a high level of expertise in the operator, coupled with only a marginal gain in sensitivity and lower specificity, TRUS is now not thought to be a suitable test for initial screening. However, it remains as a diagnostic investigation for men referred from screening as well as those with symptoms, its principal contribution being its ability to obtain directed biopsies.

Sensitivity of Screening by PSA and DRE Combined

Working on the basis of findings in the American Cancer Society study [32] in which all three tests were used but PSA levels were only acted upon if over 10 ng/ml and if the other tests were negative, Kramer et al. [25] estimate that the relative sensitivity (i.e. using all screen-detected cancers as the denominator) of abnormal PSA (above 4 ng/ml) and/or abnormal rectal examination is 84%, the specificity 92% and the positive predictive value 18%. These levels are comparable to those obtained in screening for breast cancer by mammography (Chapter 3). This combination of tests is currently regarded as the best available procedure, saving TRUS for performing directed biopsies in men with positive findings on either PSA or DRE.

As yet no data have been published on the rate at which "interval" prostate cancers occur following a negative screen, and therefore all these estimates of sensitivity are bound to be underestimates, and there is no information on which to base decisions on the frequency with which routine screening should be repeated. Similarly there is as yet no consensus on the age at which screening should start (some advocating it as young as 40 years) nor on the age at which it should stop (some considering that early detection is only useful in men aged under 70 years [47].

Prevalence of Prostate Cancer at Screening

A wide range of prevalence has been reported reflecting the diversity of the populations in different studies. They vary according to their nationality, their age distribution, their symptom distribution, their method of recruitment and the screening tests employed. Table 7.2 illustrates some of the findings.

Table 7.2   Prevalence of prostate cancer at screening

Study	Size of sample	Age range (years)	Source of recruitment	Screening test(s)	Prevalence per 1000 screened
Mettlin et al. 1991 (USA) [32]	2425	55–70	Clinic attenders for unrelated condition	DRE + TRUS + PSA > 10 ng/ml	24
Catalona et al. 1991 (USA) [8]	1653	50+		PSA > 4 ng/ml	22
Mueller et al. 1988 (USA) [34]	4843			DRE	16.5
Chodak et al. 1989 (USA) [11]	2131		Self-referred	DRE	14.5
Pedersen, 1990 (Sweden) [38]	1494	50–69	Random selection	DRE	8.7
Chadwick et al. 1991 (UK) [9]	814	55–70	GP register	DRE + PSA > 4 ng/ml	8.5
Watanabe et al. 1989 (Japan) [53]	6529			TRUS	6.4
Faul (Germany) [14]	1 500 000	45+	Attenders for routine health-check	DRE	1.3

With the exception of the German figure [14], which comes from a system in which all men aged 45 years and over are eligible for a routine health check by a general practitioner each year, the yield of prostate cancer at screening exceeds the expected annual incidence by a factor of 6 or more. The prevalence to incidence ratio gives a rough guide to the average number of years of lead-time gained by screening – in this case 6 years or more. This high prevalence to incidence ratio suggests that screening is detecting a large proportion of very slowly progressive disease.

Acceptability of Screening

Many of the past American studies have been among volunteers or among men already receiving medical care, although not necessarily for urological conditions. Such groups are more motivated to accept screening tests than are asymptomatic men in the general population. However, in one study of over 2000 men who had self-referred for their initial digital rectal examination and who were recommended to repeat the test each year, only 63% attended for the first annual repeat, falling to 22% for the second annual repeat [11].

In the German programme, only 15% of the male population aged 45 years and over attend for the annual health check [18]. However, there is no system for routine invitations, and the health check is not permitted during a consultation for any symptomatic complaint, but requires a separate visit to the doctor. In a Swedish study in which men aged 50–69 years on a population register were invited for screening by DRE 78% accepted [38]. In a British study of screening by DRE and PSA [9] 58% of men invited from a general practice register attended for screening.

The Effect of Screening on Prostate Cancer Mortality

To date, no studies have been published which analyse the effect of screening on prostate cancer mortality. The closest is a case-control study [17] of the effect of digital rectal examination on the subsequent incidence of metastatic prostate cancer, which, because of its poor prognosis is a reasonable surrogate for mortality. This study was conducted within a health maintenance organisation (HMO) in the San Francisco Bay area, where annual screening by digital rectal examination was offered, and where good medical records of every person enrolled in the HMO were maintained. A total of 139 cases of metastatic prostate cancer were compared with an equal number of matched controls without metastatic prostate cancer, in respect of the number of digital rectal examinations they had had during the past 10 years prior to diagnosis of the case. The relative risk of metastatic prostate cancer in men who had had at least one examination compared to men who had had none was 0.9 (95% CI 0.5–1.7). This non-significant finding is compatible with either a reduction in risk of advanced cancer or an excess but suggests that the effect which availability of DRE screening will have on mortality is small. However, the average number of examinations in participants in this study was only three, over periods exceeding 10 years, so the possibility that a greater reduction in risk might have been seen if screening had been more frequent cannot be ruled out.

Another study with possibly depressing conclusions about the effectiveness of digital rectal examination as a screening test examined the 5- and 10-year disease specific survival of men with screen-detected prostate cancer [20]. The study was uncontrolled and a variety of different treatments ranging from observation to combinations of radical treatments were used. Cancer specific survival at 5 and 10 years for the whole group was 92% and 75%, respectively, but there was a significant difference between those whose cancer was detected at the first (prevalence) screen (10-year survival 86%), and those detected at subsequent annual screens (10-year survival 57%), despite the fact that the stage distribution was similar at both screens. The authors conclude that more sensitive and/or more frequent screening may be required to pick up faster growing aggressive tumours.

The uncertainty about the effect of screening on prostate cancer mortality can only be resolved by a randomised controlled trial in which men are randomised to an intervention group who are offered screening and a control group who are not; all would be followed-up for a long period to determine any difference between them in the death rate from prostate cancer.

One such trial is now in progress in the US funded by the National Cancer Institute [25]. A total of 74 000 men will be randomised; the 37 000 in the screening arm will be offered screening by PSA and DRE at entry, followed by three additional annual tests. The sample size provides 90% power to determine a 20% decrease in mortality after 10 years. Contamination of the control group due to men seeking screening will be monitored, and the sample size increased if necessary. A similar multicentre trial is currently being piloted in a number of centres in Europe [46]. Given that these studies are still only in their recruitment stage, the answer to the effectiveness of prostate cancer screening will not be known until the year 2005 at the earliest, and probably 2010.

The Potential Disadvantages of Screening for Prostate Cancer

The four principal disadvantages of screening for prostate cancer which need to be considered are the lack of specificity of current screening tests, the potential for overdiagnosis and overtreatment, the side-effects of treatment, and the costs of the screening programme and management costs arising from it.

Lack of Specificity

With current levels of specificity, up to 8% of men without prostate cancer will be subjected to anxiety about the possibility of cancer and will be required to undergo the unpleasant examination of transrectal ultrasound with several punch biopsies. Some of these men will have benign prostatic hypertrophy and it could be argued that these may benefit from early diagnosis. However, given that treatment of BPH is directed only at symptom relief, its value to men who have not yet sought relief is questionable.

Overdiagnosis

It is clear from the numerous natural history studies that very many more men have prostate cancer than are at risk of dying from it. Detection of a non-fatal prostate cancer is of no benefit and is harmful due to the anxiety it generates, and the physical morbidity associated with treatment and follow-up. Some idea of the potential for overdiagnosis can be obtained by comparing the yield of prostate cancer found at screening with the expected incidence up to age 75 or 80 years. As already noted, the prevalence to incidence ratio is at least 6; Miller [33] draws attention to a prevalence to incidence ratio of 9 in a Swedish study. Given the prolonged natural history of many prostate cancers and the probability of death from competing causes before the cancer spreads to become metastatic, over-diagnosis is a very real problem. Its extent can only be quantified by the proposed randomised controlled trials of screening, provided that both intervention group and control group are followed-up until all subjects have died.

Side-Effects of Treatment

The seriousness of overdiagnosis as a consequence of screening is accentuated in the case of prostate cancer by the fact that many patients will perforce be treated by radical prostatectomy or by radical radiotherapy, rather than by a watchful waiting policy. Lu-Yao and Greenberg [21, 31] examined radical prostatectomy rates in US areas covered by SEER cancer registries and noted that in the Seattle area the risk of having a radical prostatectomy by age 75 years was five times greater than the risk of dying from prostate cancer. Moreover, although mortality rates did not vary much over time or over different parts of the US, radical prostatectomy rates and incidence rates did; they conclude that these differences are not due to true under-lying differences in the frequency of prostate cancer but reflect the aggressiveness with which screening and radical surgery is practised in different parts of the country.

The introduction of a nerve-sparing surgical technique in radical prostatectomy has reduced the risk of impotence, one of its more serious sequelae [7]. Never-theless this extensive surgery has other serious side-effects and only a proportion of cases are eligible for the nerve-sparing operation. Greenwald et al. [21] quote an operative mortality rate of 1.2%, an impotence rate of 10%–25%, an incontinence rate of 6%, a rectal injury/colostomy rate of 3% and a urethral stricture rate of 18%. These complication rates are largely derived from clinical series in patients of whom many may have been symptomatic and possibly including men of older ages than those likely to be included in a screening programme. Nevertheless the patients in these series were clearly deemed to be "operable" and may, therefore, have had similar rates of co-morbidity to men whose cancer is detected by screen-ing.

Although radical prostatectomy is probably the most frequent treatment method for screen detected cases in the USA, others receive external beam irradiation. Com-parable complication rates of radiotherapy quoted by Greenwald et al. [21] are: treatment associated mortality 0.5%; impotence 25%; rectal injury/colostomy 1%; incontinence 3%; urethral stricture 8%.

Fleming et al. [15] have developed a Markovian model, based on published medical literature, for a decision analysis of alternative treatment strategies for clinically localised prostate cancer. This took account of complication rates to adjust for quality of life. The sensitivity of the results was tested by varying several of the parameters but this had little effect on the conclusions. It was found that in all patients over the age of 70 years, and in younger patients aged 60–65 years with well-differentiated tumours a policy of watchful waiting resulted in better quality-adjusted life-expectancy than either radical prostatectomy or radiotherapy. Only among the youngest age-group (aged under 65 years) with moderately or poorly differentiated tumours, did radical treatment improve quality-adjusted life expectancy, and there was little difference between radical prostatectomy and radiotherapy.

This theoretical analysis may be able to be validated against the prospective trials of alternative treatments [24] in the Nordic countries. However, since the latter trials are mainly in symptomatic or incidental prostate cancers, the relevance to screen-detected cancers (which may contain a proportion of apparently localised low-grade tumours subsequently destined to a more aggressive course) may be limited, and the final conclusions on quality-adjusted life expectancy resulting from screening will have to await the randomised trials of screening.

The possibility that these harmful side-effects of screening may well outweigh its potential has led some to question whether trials of screening for prostate cancer are even ethical [1].

Resource Costs

Some attempts have been made to estimate the resource costs within population screening studies. Carlsson et al. [3] used the findings of a screening programme in 50–69-year-old men, to compare the costs of no screening, with a DRE screening policy, and a DRE plus TRUS screening policy. The "benefits" of screening were expressed as the total number of potentially curative treatments which resulted. This measure differs from costs per case detected in that advanced cases were not included as benefits, but it makes the assumption that all of the early cases detected benefited from treatment, ignoring the problem of overdiagnosis. They concluded that in the whole of Sweden over a 2-year period the cost of a DRE screening policy per potentially curable man would be $US 14 249.

Littrup et al. [30] investigated the cost per cancer detected in the American Cancer Society National Prostate Cancer Detection Project which includes serum PSA in the screening procedure. They found by sensitivity analyses that the three most important determinants of cost per case detected were the specificity of screening, the difference between costs of treating advanced disease and early disease, and the prevalence of prostate cancer. This study included the cost of overdiagnosis and of complications of treatment but details of these values are not given. In looking at the individual modalities it was found that DRE in skilled hands gave the lowest cost per case detected but that a minor decrease in skill, lowering both sensitivity and specificity, resulted in one of the most costly detection scenarios. The investigators also noted that if the cost of PSA testing (30 US dollars in their study) could be reduced as is likely with automation and centralisation of laboratories, this could have a major impact on costs.

However, these attempts to develop some measure of the cost-effectiveness of screening for prostate cancer acknowledge the central difficulty that as yet the effectiveness of prostate cancer screening in reducing mortality has not been measured. No doubt an economic analysis will be performed within the current US National Cancer Institute randomised controlled trial.

Conclusions

Screening for prostate cancer, although widely practised in the USA is more controversial than screening for many other common cancer sites. The increasing incidence of prostate cancer in the US is sometimes cited as a reason for introducing screening as a means of control. But screening exacerbates increasing incidence rather than controlling it, and apparently has led to very many men being subjected to radical treatment, some of whom suffer or even die from its side-effects.

Screening is intended to control mortality but, as yet, there is no evidence of the proportion of deaths which could be prevented. The acceptability of repeated screening which includes digital rectal examinations is low in many studies, and the combination of PSA and DRE is not very sensitive, particularly when one remembers that no studies have so far reported on interval cancer rates. Any potential for early detection to reduce mortality will be limited by these factors.

The elderly age and co-morbidity of men in the prostate cancer age band, the exceedingly slow progression of a majority of prostate cancers, and the serious side-effects of treatment mean that there is a real possibility that screening could be doing more harm than good. Unless and until the randomised controlled trials of screening, which are now starting, show otherwise, there is no case for population screening for prostate cancer.

References

1. Adami H-O, Baron JA, Rothman KJ (1994) Ethics of a prostate cancer screening trial. Lancet 343:958–960.
2. Armbruster DA (1993) Prostate specific antigen: biochemistry, analytical methods and clinical application. Clin Chem 39:181–185.
3. Carlsson P, Pedersen KV, Varenhorst E (1990) Costs and benefits of early detection of prostatic cancer. Health Policy 16:241–253.
4. Carter BS, Carter HB, Isaacs JT (1990) Epidemiologic evidence regarding predisposing factors to prostate cancer. Prostate 16:187–197.
5. Carter BS, Beaty TH, Steinberg GD, Childs B, Walsh PC (1992) Mendelian inheritance of familial prostate cancer. Proc Natl Acad Sci USA 89:3367–3371.
6. Carter HB, Pearson JD, Metter EJ et al. (1992) Longitudinal evaluation of prostate-specific antigen. Levels in men with and without prostate disease. JAMA 267:2215–

2220.

7. Catalona WJ (1990) Patient selection for, results of, and impact on tumour resection of potency-sparing radical prostatectomy. Urol Clin North Am 17:819–826.

8. Catalona WJ, Smith DS, Ratcliffe TL et al. (1991) Measurement of prostate specific antigen in serum as a screening test for prostate cancer. N Engl J Med 324:1156–1161.

9. Chadwick DJ, Kemple T, Astley JP et al. (1991) Pilot study of screening for prostate cancer in general practice. Lancet 338:613–616.

10. Chisholm GD (1981) Perspectives and prospects. In: Duncan W (ed) Recent results in cancer research. Prostate cancer. Springer, Berlin, pp 173–184.

11. Chodak GW, Keller P, Schoenberg HW (1989) Assessment of screening for prostate cancer using the digital rectal examination. J Urol 141:1136–1138.

12. Coleman MP, Esteve J, Damiecki P et al. (1993) Trends in cancer incidence and mortality. IARC Sci Publ 121. IARC, Lyon.

13. Cooner WH, Mosley BR, Rutherford CL et al. (1988) Clinical application of transrectal ultrasonography and prostate-specific antigen in the search for prostate cancer. J Urol 139:758.

14. Faul P (1982) Experience with the German annual preventive check-up examination. In: Jacobi GH, Hohenfellner R (eds) Prostate cancer. Williams and Wilkins, Baltimore, pp 57–70.

15. Fleming C, Wasson JH, Albertsen PC, Barry MJ, Wennberg JE (1993) A decision analysis of alternative treatment strategies for clinically localized prostate cancer. JAMA 269:2650–2657.

16. Franks LM (1954) Latent carcinoma of the prostate. J Pathol Bacteriol: 68: 603–616.

17. Friedman GD, Hiath RA, Queensbury CP, Selby JV (1991) Case-control study of screening for prostatic cancer by digital rectal examinations. Lancet 337:1526–1529.

18. Frohmuller H (1991) Screening for prostatic cancer. The German experience. Acta Oncol 30:269–272.

19. George NJR (1988) Natural history of localised prostatic cancer managed by conservative therapy alone. Lancet i:105–124.

20. Gerber GS, Thompson IM, Thisted R, Chodak GW (1993) Disease-specific survival following routine prostate cancer screening by digital rectal examination. JAMA 269:61–64.

21. Greenwald P, Kramer B, Weed D (1993) Expanding horizons in breast and prostate cancer prevention and early detection. J Cancer Educ 8:91–107.

22. Hanks GE (1991) Radiotherapy or surgery for prostate cancer. Acta Oncol 30:231–237.

23. Hoare IA, Alexander RL (1991) A survey of the reference limits for prostate specific antigen in apparently healthy males age 40–86 years. Clin Chem 37:1054.

24. Johannson J-E, Adami H-O, Andersson S-O, Bergstrom R, Holmberg L, Krusemo UB (1992) High 10-year survival rate in patients with early untreated prostatic cancer. JAMA 267:2191–2196.

25. Kramer BS, Brown ML, Prorok PC, Potosky AL, Gohagen JK (1993) Prostate cancer screening: what we know and what we need to know. Ann Intern Med 119:914–923.

26. Lange PH, Brawer MK (1989) Serum prostate specific antigen; its use in diagnosis and management of prostate cancer. Urology 33 (Suppl):13–19.

27. Leandri P, Rossignol G, Gautier J-R, Ramon J (1992) Radical retropubic prostatectomy: morbidity and quality of life. Experience with 620 consecutive cases. J Urol 149:883–887.

28. Lee F, Littrup PJ, Torp-Pederson ST et al. (1988) Comparison of transrectal US and digital rectal examination for screening. Radiology 168:389–394.

29. Lineham WM (1992) Molecular genetics of tumour suppressor genes in prostate carcinoma: the challenge and the promise ahead. J Urol 147:808–809.

30. Littrup PJ, Goodman AC, Mettlin C (1993) The benefit and cost of prostate cancer early detection. CA 43:134–149.

31. Lu-Yao GL, Greenberg ER (1994) Changes in prostate cancer incidence and treatment in USA. Lancet 343:251–254.

32. Mettlin C, Lee F, Drago J, Murphy GP and Investigators of the American Cancer Society National Prostate Cancer Detection Project (1991) Findings on the detection of early prostate cancer in 2425 men. Cancer 67: 2949–2958.

33. Miller AB (1991) Issues in screening for prostate cancer. In: Miller AB, Chamberlain J, Day NE, Hakama M, Prorok P (eds) Cancer screening. Cambridge University Press, Cambridge, pp 289–293.

34. Mueller EJ, Crain TW, Thompson IM, Rodriguez FR (1988) An evaluation of serial digital rectal examinations in screening for prostate cancer. J Urol 140:1445–1447.

35. Muir CS, Nectoux J, Staszewski J (1991) The epidemiology of prostatic cancer. Geographical distribution and time-trends. Acta Oncol 30:133–140.

36. Office of Population Censuses and Surveys (1993) Cancer statistics, 1987, Series MBI, No. 20. HMSO, London.

37. Office of Population Censuses and Surveys (1993) Mortality statistics, 1992 Series DH2 No. 19. HMSO, London.

38. Pedersen KV, Carlsson P, Varenhorst E, Lofman O, Berglund K (1990) Screening for carcinoma of the prostate by digital rectal examination in a randomly selected population. Br Med J 300:1041–1044.

39. Potosky AR, Kessler L, Gridley G, Brown CC, Horm JW (1990) Rise in prostatic cancer incidence associated with increased use of transurethral resection. J Natl Cancer Inst 82:1624–1627.

40. Resnick MI (1992) Staging. J Urol 147:881–882.

41. Rich AR (1935) On the frequency of occurrence of occult carcinoma of the prostate. J Urol 33:215–223.

42. Roetzheim RG, Herold AH (1992) Prostate cancer screening. Prim Care 3:637–649.

43. Rooney C, Beral V, Maconochie N, Fraser P, Davies G (1993) Case-control study of prostatic cancer in employees of the United Kingdom Atomic Energy Authority. Br Med J 307:1391–1397.

44. Schmid H-P, McNeal JE, Stamey TA (1993) Observations on the doubling time of prostate cancer. Cancer 71:2031–2040.

45. Schmidt JD, Mettlin C, Natarajan N et al. (1986) Trends in patterns of care of prostate cancer, 1973–1983: Results of surveys by the American College of Surgeons. J Urol 136:416–421.

46. Schroder FH (1993) Prostate cancer: to screen or not to screen? Br Med J 306:407–408.

47. Stamey TA, Kabalin JN, McNeal JE et al. (1989) Prostate specific antigen in the diagnosis and treatment of adeno-carcinoma of the prostate. J Urol 141:1076–1083.

48. Steinberg GD, Carter BS, Beaty TH, Childs B, Walsh PC (1990) Family history and the risk of prostate cancer. Prostate 17:337–347.

49. Terris MK, McNeal JE, Stamey TA (1992) Estimation of prostate cancer volume by transrectal ultrasound imaging. J Urol 147:855–877.

50. Thompson IM, Rounder JB, Teague JL et al. (1987) Impact of routine screening for adenocarcinoma of the prostate on stage distribution. J Urol 137:424.

51. Vallancien G, Prapotnich D, Sibert L et al. (1989) Comparison of the efficacy of digital rectal examination and ultrasonography in the diagnosis of prostatic cancer. Eur Urol

16:321–324.

52. Waaler G, Ludvigsen TC, Stenwig AE (1990) Prognosis of incidental prostate cancer in Aust-Agder County, Norway. Eur Urol 18:179–183.
53. Watanabe H (1989) History and applications of transrectal sonography of the prostate. Urol Clin North Am 16:617–622.
54. Whitemore AS, Keller JB, Betensky R (1991) Low-grade latent prostate cancer volume: predictor of clinical cancer incidence. J Natl Cancer Inst 83:1231–1235.
55. Wilson JM, Kemp IW, Stein GJ (1984) Do younger men have a poorer survival rate? Lancet 343:251–254.
56. Yatani R, Chigusa I, Akazaki K, Stemmermann GN, Welsh RA, Correa P (1982) Geographic pathology of latent prostatic carcinoma. Int J Cancer 29: 611–616.

8 – Screening for Cancers of Other Sites: Lung, Stomach, Oral and Neuroblastoma

Jocelyn Chamberlain

Introduction

Screening has been advocated as a means of control for various other cancer sites, four of which are reviewed here. Lung cancer, although theoretically preventable, is still the commonest cancer in the developed world and is rapidly increasing in developing countries. Studies of screening, however, have led to the conclusion that it is largely ineffective due to the rapid progression of potentially fatal disease.

Stomach cancer screening has been widely implemented in Japan where it is particularly common. In most of the rest of the world, however, screening does not have a high priority, partly because of the rapidly falling incidence in many countries, but also because of scepticism about its cost-effectiveness.

The only childhood cancer for which screening is practised is neuroblastoma, and again, a national programme has been in force in Japan for many years. However, there is increasing doubt about the ability of screening to detect the important progressive cancers, and increasing unease about overdiagnosis and overtreatment of neoplasia which would otherwise regress.

Finally, oral cancer is an important problem both in Asia where it is extremely common and in Western countries where its frequency is increasing. Research into screening for oral cancer and precancer is, however, in its infancy and its value is therefore still uncertain.

Lung Cancer

Lung cancer is by far the most important cancer problem in the developed world, and, with increasing cigarette consumption, likely to become so also in the developing world. In England and Wales there were 36 275 newly registered cases in 1987 [59] and 34 190 deaths in 1992 [60]. In men, lung cancer accounts for over 30% of cancer deaths being nearly three times commoner than prostate or colorectal cancer death. In women, lung cancer accounts for 16% of cancer deaths still being less common than breast cancer although in Scotland, and in the US, it has already overtaken breast cancer as the leading cause of cancer death. In the UK lung cancer incidence and mortality rates in men increased rapidly from 1920 onwards reaching a peak in the early 1970s, since when they have levelled off and are now beginning to decline. In women, the start of the increase was some 20 years later in the 1940s and age-specific mortality is still rising in older women although it has begun to fall in those under 55 years. These trends mirror trends in cigarette consumption some 20 years earlier [23]. The standardised registration ratio for men in 1987 was 15% lower than that 10 years earlier, but for women was nearly 30% higher [59]. In both sexes incidence rates rise steeply with increasing age, starting at about age 40 years.

Aetiology

The association between lung cancer and cigarette smoking has been firmly established by a plethora of epidemiological studies going back over a 40-year time period [65]. Cigarette smoking is associated with some 90% of lung cancer cases. Other aetiological factors include occupational exposure to asbestos, and to a number of metallic compounds. Environmental ionising radiation is also implicated, and the level of radon gas emanating from underlying rock in well insulated modern houses is increasingly recognised to raise the risk of lung cancer. Smoking acts synergistically with occupational and environmental exposures.

The strong connection with smoking means that lung cancer is, in theory, the most preventable of all cancers. However, progress in primary prevention has been slow, with legislative restrictions and disincentives to smoking probably having a greater effect than health education or medical advice. Nevertheless smoking levels have fallen, especially in men [19].

Staging, Survival and Natural History

Four main histological types of lung cancer are identified, namely squamous cell carcinoma (50%), small cell carcinoma (25%), adenocarcinoma (15%) and large cell carcinoma (10%). From the viewpoint of behaviour however, they are aggregated into small-cell and non-small-cell carcinomas, the former having very high malignant potential, the latter slightly less so. Molecular genetic studies of lung cancer, reviewed by Birrer and Brown [9], have found mutations or amplification in several oncogenes including members of the *ras*, *myc* and *erb* B families, and *Rb* and *p53* tumour suppressor genes. Some, but not all of the mutations, seem to be specific to particular cell types. It is not yet known whether these genetic changes represent successive carcinogenic "hits", nor whether they happen in an obligatory order for carcinogenesis to occur.

Stage I and II non-small cell tumours (i.e. situated more than 2 cm from the carina with or without ipsilateral hilar node involvement) may be treated by curative surgical resection, with a 5-year survival of 50% for Stage I and 25% for Stage II [81]. For later Stages only palliative treatment (mainly radiotherapy) is possible. Over 50% of patients with non-small-cell lung cancer already have metastatic disease at the time of presentation.

For small-cell lung cancers the situation is even more gloomy, the great majority presenting with metastatic disease. However, unlike non-small-cell types, these tumours are sensitive to many chemotherapeutic agents and patients with limited disease treated by chemotherapy usually achieve a temporary response, with up to 20% surviving 2 years, but there are very few long-term survivors.

The poor prognosis for lung cancer leads one to question whether there is a detectable preclinical phase in its natural history, of sufficiently long duration to enable detection of most cancers by screening.

Carcinoma in situ has been found to be prevalent in the lungs of people who have died from unrelated causes, and to be much more common in smokers than non-smokers [1].

Serial cytological studies of sputum in men working in the uranium industry showed progression from regular squamous cell metaplasia to mild moderate and severe atypia to carcinoma in situ and invasive cancer [72]. The proportion of in situ lesions which progress to invasive cancer, and the distribution of time over which they do so is not known. In screening studies which have included sputum cytology (reviewed below), the tumours detected by this method have been almost entirely squamous-cell type. The time to progression may be shorter for the more malignant forms.

Serial radiographs showing visible masses which subsequently turn out to be cancer have been used to measure rates of progression, one such study indicating a mean doubling time of 4.3 months and median lead time gained by screening of 11.7 months [95]. However, by the time a cancer reaches the stage of radiological visibility, its growth rate, if Gompertzian, may be different from what it was in an earlier phase of its history.

Mathematical models, based on data from screening studies, have also been used to estimate the mean duration of the detectable preclinical phase [28, 91]. Walter et al. [91] conclude that the average duration is 0.7 years, and that, assuming an exponential distribution and 100% sensitivity of the screening test, only 25% of lung cancers (all cell types) have detectable preclinical durations longer than 1 year, and only 6% longer than 2 years. Such estimates indicate that for screening to have any substantial effect on mortality it would need to be routinely repeated at very short intervals.

The Screening Tests

Chest radiographs and sputum cytology have been used, separately and in combination in a number of screening studies going back over the past 25 years. Two early studies in England [15, 56] used the mass radiography system, which had been established for control of tuberculosis, to screen men for lung cancer and found that chest radiograph had a sensitivity of about 55%. Three linked studies in the USA [6] compared screening by chest radiograph alone with screening by X-ray plus sputum cytology. In the dual test group, at the prevalent round, 93 out of 160 screen-detected cancers (58%) were found by X-ray alone, 37 (23%) by cytology alone and only 30 (19%) were positive to both tests. Among these prevalent cases, only 10% were small-cell type and none of these were positive on cytology [6]. There is little information available on false positive results, from which to judge the specificity of screening or the positive predictive value of each test.

Effectiveness of Screening

Several trials have examined the effect of lung cancer screening on mortality. The earliest was that of Brett [15] who, in 1959, randomised 119 industrial units employing men aged over 40 years into an intervention group, and a control group. Both groups were offered an initial X-ray and a final X-ray after 3 years, but the intervention group also received 6-monthly X-rays. More cases were operable in the intervention group (43.6%) than the control group (29%), but after 3 years there was no significant difference in the lung cancer mortality rate (0.7 per 1000 men in the intervention group and 0.8 per 1000 controls). The sample size in this study was large – more than 54 000 men – but with hindsight, it seems a pity that follow-up was not continued for longer.

In the 1970s, three large randomised controlled trials were started in the United States [6]. Two of these were designed to investigate whether sputum cytology in addition to chest radiograph resulted in lower mortality. The third, the Mayo Lung Project [29], was designed to show whether screening by X-ray and sputum cytology resulted in lower mortality than routine advice to have an annual check-up. Men at high risk of lung cancer by virtue of their age (45 years and over) and smoking habit (20 or more cigarettes per day) all underwent a prevalence screen. Those without lung cancer, and who were judged to have a life expectancy of at least 5 years were randomised into a screened group of 4618 men and a control group of 4593. The screened group were offered chest radiograph and sputum cytology every 4 months for 6 years and 75% complied. The control group were advised to have yearly chest X-rays and were contacted by mail each year.

During the study 5.5 lung cancers were diagnosed per 1000 men in the screened group compared with 3.3 per 1000 in the controls. Within the 206 study group cancers as a whole (screen-detected plus interval cases) 46% were resectable, compared with 32% of the 160 control group lung cancers. The 5-year survival rate of study group cases was 35% compared with 15% for the controls. But at the end of the 7-year study there was no significant difference in lung cancer mortality, 3.2 per 1000 screened group man-years and 3.0 per 1000 control group man-years. The results of this study provide a classic example of how optimistic early findings do not necessarily translate into real benefit, reinforcing the principles of evaluation outlined in Chapter 1, that a reduction in risk of death in the whole population is the only valid outcome measure of the effectiveness of screening. However, any potential benefit from the prevalence screen could not be measured (both groups being equal in this respect), the fact that the control group was "contaminated" by advice to be screened each year, and the relatively small sample size [71] mean that the conclusion of this trial on its own cannot be taken as proof of ineffectiveness.

The two other American trials, which did not have unscreened control groups, both found that lung cancer mortality did not differ between those screened by X-ray with cytology and those screened by X-ray alone [51, 86].

Another randomised controlled trial was started in Czechoslovakia in 1976, with a similar but more complicated design [45]. Following a general health survey, at which prevalent cases of lung cancer were identified, 6364 men aged over 40 years, who were smokers, and who were known to be free from lung cancer, were randomised into a group of 3172 who were offered 6-monthly radiological and cytological screening, and a control group of 3174. Men in the control group were screened again at the end of 3 years, and then both study and control groups were screened by X-ray only each year for a further 3 years. During the first 3 years more cancers were detected in the screened group and more were resectable, but at the end of the study there were more lung cancer deaths in the screened group (85) than the control group (67) although this difference was not statistically significant.

Two case-control studies of the efficacy of lung cancer screening have been published. The first [25] was conducted in the early 1980s in the German Democratic Republic where a 2-yearly chest radiography programme had been in operation for many years. The screening history of 130 men who had died from lung cancer when aged less than 70 years was compared with that of 260 age matched controls, half from population files and half from hospital patients. Three-quarters of cases and of controls had had at least one screen in the 2-year period preceding diagnosis. Smoking history, which was known for the hospital controls, was not correlated with screening history for either cases or controls. The odds ratio of a screened person dying from lung cancer compared to an unscreened person was 0.9 for population controls and 1.1 for hospital controls with 95% confidence intervals of 0.5–1.5 and 0.7–1.8, respectively. There was no trend according to the number of tests performed nor the interval since last test. Thus this study agrees with the randomised trials that screening has no effect on mortality.

The second case-control study is the only research which hints that screening may be having an effect [80]. It was conducted in 50 Japanese municipalities where X-ray and cytology screening had been available for many years. The screening histories of 273 men and women who had died from lung cancer when aged 40–74 years were compared with those of 1269 controls. A non-significant protective effect of screening was found (OR 0.72, 95% CI 0.5–1.03, $p = 0.07$). The possibility of selection bias accounting for any differences in this study cannot be ruled out, although the controls were matched not only for age and sex but also for smoking status and type of health insurance.

Disadvantages

The main disadvantages of lung cancer screening are overdiagnosis of cancers that would not otherwise surface in the individual's lifetime, and false positive screening results requiring expensive and possibly dangerous diagnostic work-up. Eddy [26] estimates that up to 1% of individuals might be "overdiagnosed" each year (although not specifying whether this applies when screening is carried out 4-monthly, 6-monthly or annually). From the early results of the NCI Cooperative Lung Group studies he also estimates that 10% of people undergoing X-ray and 1% of those undergoing sputum cytology will have a false positive result. For many of these subjects close surveillance is the method of management but, for some, more invasive diagnostic procedures may be required including bronchoscopy or even thoracotomy. Location of the source of a cytological abnormality when there are no radiological signs is a particular problem.

Bailar [3] noted that following the prevalence screen in the NCI Cooperative Lung Project there were two postoperative deaths in men who did not in fact have cancer. Postoperative deaths occurred in 5% of lung cancers in the Mayo project and were equally common in screened and control groups [29]. In the screened group, who would not otherwise have come to surgery until some time later, if at all, the date of death had been advanced by screening such cases.

Conclusions

There is little or no dissent from the view that screening for lung cancer cannot be recommended. Eddy [26] emphasises that this conclusion is not based on *lack* of evidence of an effect, but on consistent evidence that there is *no* effect. However, this evidence comes from studies, none of which included a completely unscreened control group, and which were either too small or too short to have statistical power for detection of a mortality reduction less than about 40% [71]. Therefore the proposed PLC trial in the USA is to be welcomed, although a comparison of annual screening chest radiographs with "usual medical care" in a society where chest X-radiographs are already so common seems likely to suffer from almost as much contamination as the existing evidence.

Stomach

Worldwide, stomach cancer is the second commonest cancer (after lung) but its frequency is declining [63]. In England and Wales the standardised registration ratio fell by 15% in males and 20% in females between 1979 and 1989 [59]. In 1987 there were 6484 registrations in men and 4271 in women, whereas mortality data [60] show that in 1992 there were 4994 and 3291 deaths, respectively. About 76% of new cases and 82% of deaths are in people aged over 65 years.

Worldwide the highest recorded incidence rates occur in Japan and parts of China, and it is also common in Latin America and in Eastern Europe. There are marked differences according to socio-economic group, rates being almost 3 times higher in unskilled than in professional classes.

Various dietary factors have been investigated as aetiological agents, including high intake of salt and of nitrates, which lead to the formation of potentially carcinogenic N-nitroso compounds in the stomach. Several case-control studies have found increased risk of stomach cancer associated with higher consumption of nitrate-containing preserved meats and cured fish and pickles, and some, but not all, studies have reported a positive association with salt intake (reviewed by Miller [52]). There is greater agreement about the protective effect of fresh fruit and vegetables and vitamin C. In recent years chronic infection with *Helicobacter pylori* is increasingly recognised to be an important cause of gastric cancer [27], accounting for some of its associations such as that with social class and poor housing [4]. Persistent *H. pylori* infection induces several mutagenic processes and DNA damage. It is thought that chronic gastritis leads to atrophy and metaplasia which are precursors of gastric cancer. Antibiotic treatment of *Helicobacter* has been suggested as a method of primary prevention [31] but is expensive and carries the risk of increasing the number of resistant strains.

Natural History, Treatment and Survival

Intestinal metaplasia of the gastric epithelium is recognised to be a precursor lesion, leading to severe dysplasia [54] and eventually invasive cancer. Early gastric cancer is defined as tumour confined to the mucosa or submucosa regardless of lymph node status and thus includes TNM Stages I and part of II. A Japanese study of 56 patients with endoscopically diagnosed early gastric cancer in whom treatment was delayed found that over an average period of 29 months, 27 progressed to advanced cancer, 16 remained the same and 13 had no further examination to determine their status [88]. Of 34 patients who did not undergo surgery, 12 died of gastric cancer.

All early stage patients are eligible for treatment by curative resection, and this form of management may also be used for patients in Stages II and III whose tumour does not involve contiguous structures and who do not have metastases. Five-year survival following radical potentially curative resection is as high as 71%, and for Stage I cancer it is 93% [85]. But a majority of patients still present with advanced disease.

Overall survival has not altered much among all registered cases in England and Wales diagnosed up to 1981 [59] and in Scotland up to 1987 [10], 5-year relative survival still being only around 10%. However, there has been an improvement in survival among patients diagnosed under the age of 65 years.

In some UK centres a recent trend towards earlier presentation has been reported; for example, one study reported the proportion of cases in whom potentially curative resection was possible increased from 30% in 1970 to 55% in 1989, and the proportion with Stage I disease increased from 4% to 26% in the same time period [85]. The authors attribute this favourable trend to increasing use of endoscopy and biopsy for investigation of dyspeptic symptoms. But this series was hospital-based rather than population-based and therefore selection bias in changing criteria of referral to the centre cannot be ruled out as part of the explanation.

Screening Tests

The three screening methods which have been tried are double-contrast barium radiograph, tumour markers, and symptom questionnaires, followed up by endoscopy.

Double contrast barium radiography has been provided as a screening service in Japan for over 30 years. Although all people over age 40 years are eligible, participation has been very low, increasing from 8% in 1984 to 13% in 1990 [92]. There is little information about its sensitivity, although one paper from Miyagi Prefecture states that sensitivity (using the conventional method of estimation) is 85% [38]. However, its main disadvantage is lack of specificity, a level of only 90% meaning that nearly 10% of screened subjects have to undergo further diagnostic tests. The predictive value of a positive test is only 1.7%.

The validity of *tumour markers* in screening for stomach cancer has been studied in Finland, which has a high incidence. The level of fetal sulphoglycoprotein antigen in gastric juice was used in one population screening programme in which, at one year sensitivity was 75%, falling to 47% at 3 years; specificity was also low, at 91% [33]. Subsequently a serum bank was used to undertake a nested case-control study of the validity of a number of tumour markers in serum for identification of subsequent gastrointestinal cancers [34]. The best marker for stomach cancer, CA 19–9, had a sensitivity of 73%, but a very low specificity of 74% making it inapplicable for population screening.

Presence of dyspepsia symptoms has not been studied as a primary screening test among people who have not previously complained. It was noted in one study

[35] involving a population of 45 000 subjects aged over 45 years, that over a four-year period 2659 people (5.9%) were referred by their general practitioner for endoscopic investigation of dyspeptic symptoms. A total of 57 gastric cancers were found (positive predictive value 2%) and a further 493 (19%) patients had high risk conditions of the gastric mucosa and were kept under annual endoscopic surveillance. Potentially curative surgery was possible in 36 of the patients with gastric cancer (63%) and, among these 15 cases (26%) were classified as "early". Sensitivity and specificity cannot be derived from this study since nothing is known about the 94% of the population who were not referred.

Effectiveness of Screening

The most relevant evidence comes from Japan where mass screening by double-contrast barium radiography has been provided since 1962, when it was introduced, unfortunately without a randomised controlled trial. Although a vast experience of screening has been obtained, the generally low participation rate already referred to hinders attempts to quantify the effect of screening on gastric cancer mortality.

Gastric cancer mortality has been falling in Japan since the introduction of screening, but over the same time period there have been changes in diet and improvements in living standards both of which must have contributed substantially to a lower incidence of the disease. In Miyagi Prefecture which has had a population based cancer registry since 1952, incidence rates and mortality rates declined in parallel between 1960 and 1970, but since then mortality has been declining more quickly than incidence. The increasing separation between the rates is attributed in part to screening, although other explanations such as improved therapy, and improved ascertainment of cases by the cancer registry cannot be ruled out [38]. When trends in stage-specific incidence are examined there has been an increase in the rate of early cancer, and a decline in the incidence of advanced cancer.

Case-control studies have also been used to evaluate the Japanese programme. Oshima et al. [61] undertook a study which included as cases all 91 stomach cancer deaths between 1969 and 1981 in the town of Nose. Three controls, matched for age and area of residence, were randomly selected for each case, and the screening histories of cases and controls up to the date of diagnosis of the case were compared. When tests conducted in the 12 months preceding diagnosis (i.e. those which might have been for investigation of symptoms) were ignored, the odds ratio of a screened person dying of stomach cancer compared with an unscreened person was 0.519 for men and 0.486 for women, both findings being significant at the 5% level. Another case-control study [30] took patients with advanced cancer diagnosed by screening as cases, matched each with one control from the screening register, and then examined different time intervals since the last negative screen. This methodology cannot provide information on the effectiveness of screening versus not screening, but shows how protection falls off with increasing time since last screen. It was concluded that screening should be repeated at intervals no greater than 3 years. However, a third case-control study in Venezuela found no conclusive evidence of benefit, a finding which is attributed to the tendency of symptomatic subjects to self-refer for screening [68].

A theoretical model was used to estimate the cost-effectiveness of screening in Japan from which it was calculated that in 1990 the screening programme cost

$US 55 000 for each life saved [38]. It is reasonable to conclude that although screening by double contrast barium radiograph may confer some benefit, it is only feasible in a country with a high stomach cancer mortality rate and plentiful resources.

Neuroblastoma

Neuroblastoma is the only childhood cancer for which screening has yet been tried. It is a tumour of embryonal cells in the neural crest and may arise in the medulla of the suprarenal gland or elsewhere along the sympathetic nervous system from the neck to the pelvis.

Data from childhood cancer registries [84] show that its incidence, at least in Western Europe, has been increasing over the past 20 years particularly at young ages. But worldwide there is little variation [64], with a cumulative incidence up to age 15 years of 1-1.4 per 10 000 live-births. During the course of childhood, incidence falls with increasing age from 30 per million in infants under age 1 year, down to less than one per million in children aged 10-14 years [24]. Mortality data are not routinely available because the International Classification of Diseases does not have a specific code for neuroblastoma. But cancer registries which routinely receive malignant disease death notifications in childhood are able to produce mortality statistics. In the UK, mortality fell steadily during the 1970s despite increasing incidence, but the fall has been less steep in recent years. During the period 1983-87 about four children per million died from neuroblastoma each year in the UK [84].

Case-fatality data confirm the fact that treatment has contributed to lower mortality. The UK 5-year survival rate has improved from 15% among cases diagnosed in the early 1970s to 43% in 1983-85 [83]. More recent data from Scandinavia [73] and North America [7] show survival rates over 50%. As with other childhood tumours improvements in chemotherapy account for the trend but nevertheless the prognosis for neuroblastoma has not improved to the same extent as that of other solid tumours in childhood.

Prognosis is dependent not only on stage, but also, independently, on age at diagnosis, younger children with advanced disease faring better than their older counterparts [22]. The staging system for neuroblastoma [17] includes an unusual category of Stage IVS (S for special). Tumours at this stage, which by definition occur only in infants under 1 year, have a unilateral localised primary but appear to have massive metastatic involvement of the liver and sometimes bone marrow; nevertheless these infants have an excellent prognosis and some cases may even regress without therapy [44]. True Stage IV disease, however, with disseminated primary tumour and widespread metastases, has a very poor prognosis with a 5-year survival rate of 20% or less.

Natural History

Neuroblastoma is a disease with a very variable natural history. Autopsy studies of the adrenal glands of fetuses and infants who have died of other conditions before the age of 3 months, show that in situ neuroblastomas are present in as many as 1 in 250 infants [5]. This prevalence is about 40 times greater than the cumulative lifetime incidence of clinical neuroblastoma, indicating that spontaneous regression occurs in a majority of these in situ cases.

The range of malignancy of clinical neuroblastomas is increasingly being elucidated by various biological markers. Neuroblastomas secrete catecholamines and their metabolites are excreted in the urine of the patients. Abnormal levels of homovanillic acid (HVA) and vanillyl mandelic acid (VMA) are found in 93% of clinical cases, and it has been shown that an HVA to VMA ratio greater than 1 is associated with a poor prognosis [90]. Two genetic changes found in poor prognosis tumours are deletion or translocation of the 1p zone on the short arm of chromosome 1 [37], and amplification of the *n-myc* oncogene [16]. These prognostic features within a given tumour do not change over time, and thus there is little support for the concept of phenotypic drift accounting for the observation that prognosis becomes worse with increasing age at diagnosis.

The Screening Test

Urinary levels of catecholamine metabolites form the basis for the screening test, which is usually performed at about 6 months of age. It has been found feasible to obtain sufficient urine for testing by blotting a wet nappy (diaper) onto a filter paper, which is then sent to a laboratory for testing. HVA and VMA levels are measured in terms of μg/mg of creatinine using either high performance liquid chromatography or gas chromatography with mass spectrometry. Because of variation with age and interlaboratory variations in these assays the cut-off level between normal and suspicious is taken to be two standard deviations above the mean level of either metabolite for that age tested in that laboratory. If either metabolite is above this level the test is repeated, using a second punched-out sample from the same filter-paper; if the level is three standard deviations above the mean then the child is referred for clinical examination. In practice, less than 1 in 1000 infants are referred giving the test a very high level of specificity.

Test sensitivity is judged by the number of symptomatic interval cancers arising after a negative screen. Since the test at 6 months is intended to detect all the neuroblastomas which would otherwise present throughout childhood, recording the number of interval cancers requires a follow-up of 10 years or even longer.

Following some early studies, Japan has had a national screening programme in operation since 1985 [76]. However, accurate data on interval cancers depend on a childhood cancer registry which is not provided nationally in Japan but only in certain prefectures. Nishi et al. [58] reported that six interval cancers were diagnosed after screening 120 170 infants among whom 22 neuroblastomas were detected, from which they concluded that sensitivity was 78% (22/28); however, the period of follow-up was not stated. In a British study [62] three interval cancers were diagnosed during a period of 2½ years after screening 22 100 infants among who two neuroblastomas were screen-detected, giving a sensitivity of only 40%. In Canada, where screening is carried out at 3 weeks of age, four neuroblastomas were detected in 41 673 infants, and one interval case subsequently presented giving a sensitivity of 80%. Clearly in such a rare condition there is a problem in drawing statistically valid conclusions from very small numbers. It would be preferable to express sensitivity by the proportional incidence method (the proportion of the expected incidence of neuroblastomas in successive periods after screening which present as interval cancers) but the period of follow-up is only stated in the British study.

An analysis of prognostic features of neuroblastomas in the Japanese programme [41] showed that screen-detected cases tended to be relatively benign, whereas interval cases were of higher malignancy. It may be that screening in infancy is not able to detect the poor prognosis cases which must be caught early if screening is to have an effect [96].

The Benefits of Screening

The purpose of screening in infancy is to detect and treat a high proportion of the neuroblastomas which would otherwise present at an advanced stage in older children. Therefore its benefits should be seen firstly in a reduction in the incidence of neuroblastoma at older ages and secondly in a reduction in deaths.

Some of the early reports from Japan compared the proportion of cases diagnosed under age 1 year before and after the introduction of screening [74] or in screened areas versus unscreened areas [57] and concluded that screening was having an effect. However, more cases diagnosed under age 1 year does not necessarily mean that fewer cases were being diagnosed at later ages. From data presented from Sapporo [57] it seems that, before screening, the average annual number of cases in children over the age of 1 year was 2.7, falling to 2 per year after the introduction of screening; however, no data are given about changes in the size or age-distribution of the child population. Subsequently an analysis of data from a hospital-based cancer registry subtracted screen-detected neuroblastomas from the remainder and then found no change in the percentage age distribution of neuroblastomas during a 5-year period after the introduction of screening compared with that before [8]. The implication of this is that screening is detecting biologically benign tumours which would not otherwise present and failing to detect those destined to present at later ages.

One clinical series, which included only about two-thirds of neuroblastomas diagnosed in the relevant population presented a contrary view [55]. After the introduction of screening it was noted that fewer children over the age of 1 year were presenting, and that the difference was most marked in the third year of life. The same paper pointed out that 5-year survival improved from 23% in cases diagnosed in 1972–80 to 67% in cases diagnosed in 1981–89; 27 out of 50 cases in the latter period were detected by screening. But although this series is consistent with a screening benefit it is not conclusive, firstly because it does not include all cases in the population, secondly because the change in survival coincided with the period when chemotherapy was having its principal impact, and thirdly because no allowance was made for lead-time bias, length-biased sampling and overdiagnosis among the cases detected by screening. Similar doubts apply to Sawada et al.'s [76] report that in 1990, 328 (97%) of 337 screen-detected cases in the whole of Japan since the start of the programme were still alive, including 78 out of 83 diagnosed at Stage III or IV.

Only one study has so far been published, which looks at population-based mortality from neuroblastoma in relation to screening [36]. Because neuroblastoma does not have a specific code in the International Classification of Diseases a laborious search was made of the case-notes of 190 children who had died in Japan between 1979 and 1987 with a certified cause of death from malignant neoplasm of the retroperitoneum, mediastinum, head and neck, thorax, abdomen and pelvis. A total of 135 neuroblastoma deaths were identified and added to the 902 deaths certified as dying from malignant neoplasm of the adrenal gland, all of which were assumed to be neuroblastoma. The neuroblastoma death rate per 100 000 population of different age-groups was then plotted over time. In children aged 1–4 years, a statistically significant 45% reduction in mortality was observed when comparing the death rate before 1985 (when screening was implemented nationally) and later. There was no significant decline in other age-groups so improvement in therapy is an unlikely explanation. However, there remains doubt about how much of the decline can be attributed to screening. Chamberlain [20] points out that the drop in mortality in children aged 1 to 4 was limited to a single year between 1984 and 1985, and children in this age-group then would have been eligible for screening during their first year between 1980 and 1984 which was before the national programme started and when less than 10% of Japanese infants were screened. A repeat of this analysis in future years, analysing mortality in cohorts of children born in different years and for which the proportion screened in their first year of life is known, would elucidate the effect of screening in Japan.

Disadvantages of Screening

The main disadvantage of neuroblastoma screening is the psychological and physical morbidity arising from overdiagnosis and treatment of tumours which would otherwise have regressed. Screen-detected cases are known to be biased towards those without n-*myc* amplification or chromosome 1p deletion, thus having an inherently good prognosis [43], and there are isolated case reports of cases managed solely by observation which have regressed [50].

Further evidence of overdiagnosis comes from a comparison of the yield of disease at screening and the expected cumulative lifetime incidence. Assuming a cumulative incidence of 14 per 100 000 (towards the upper end of the range of reported figures) the yield of neuroblastomas found at screening plus the interval cases so far reported exceeds this frequency in the UK [62], in Canada [89], and in at least one centre in Japan [75]. There is therefore little doubt that cases of disease which would otherwise regress are detected by screening and subjected to the serious side-effects of treatment, perhaps even including operative mortality in a few instances.

Conclusion

Although in theory screening for neuroblastoma should be able to save a large number of life-years, its benefits remain unproven, whereas its side-effects are serious. A large North American trial currently in progress will compare a screened population of 500 000 in Quebec with a number of unscreened populations in the United States, and aims to detect a 40% or greater reduction in mortality [7]. Unless and until this trial shows such a reduction, screening for neuroblastoma cannot be recommended.

Oral Cancer

Worldwide, cancers of the oral cavity, including the lip, tongue, and oropharynx, are the sixth commonest form of cancer [64]. However, with the exception of parts of France, they are relatively infrequent in western Europe and North America, and mainly affect an elderly age-group. In 1992 in England and Wales 903 men and 479 women died from oral cancer with 55% of new cases and 66% of deaths being among people aged over 65 years [59, 60].

A substantial reduction in oral cancer mortality occurred in developed countries up until 1970, but recently, cohort analyses demonstrate that it is again rising [13]. In the Indian subcontinent and the rest of South East Asia oral cancer is particularly common, being the leading cause of cancer and cancer death in males [49]. Because of its worldwide incidence and increasing incidence in developed countries oral cancer is a high priority for developing a means of control [14].

Aetiology

Numerous case-control studies, reviewed by Boyle et al. [13], have consistently found an increased risk in tobacco smokers, with a dose-response effect, and with an effect present in cigar smokers as well as cigarette smokers; pipe smokers have an increased risk of lip cancers. Similarly case-control studies have shown a lesser but consistent association between alcohol consumption and oral cancer which appears to be independent of smoking [40], although the two substances may act synergistically to give an even greater risk in people who both smoke and drink [12].

In South-East Asia, chewing of betel quid, which is very widespread, is the prime risk factor. There is a strong association between the risk of oral cancer and the duration of chewing, the highest risk being found among those who retain the quid in their mouths while asleep, and being most frequent at the site in the mouth where the quid is normally kept [39]. The betel quid may contain areca-nut, slaked lime and tobacco in addition to betel vine leaf, and risk is greater in those who chew betel with tobacco, and in those who both smoke and chew. A working party of the International Agency for Research on Cancer [39] concluded that there was sufficient evidence that betel quid containing tobacco is harmful but inadequate evidence on the carcinogenicity of betel quid without tobacco.

Another form of tobacco consumption, practised mainly in the southern United States is oral snuff or "snuff-dipping", pouches of tobacco being placed and retained between cheek and gum. This too has been shown to increase risk of oral cancer [47].

Other risk factors which have been investigated with less clear-cut findings are poor dental hygiene (in which chronic trauma and infection are postulated to be carcinogenic), frequent use of mouth washes (whose alcohol content may be carcinogenic) and oncogenic viruses.

A high dietary intake of fresh fruit and green leafy vegetables, with their vitamin A and vitamin C content, has been shown in several studies to be protective [48].

Natural History

Oral cancers are among those for which premalignant changes can be identified. The World Health Organization [97] defined a precancerous oral *lesion* as "a morphologically altered tissue in which oral cancer is more likely to occur than in its normal counterpart", and a precancerous *condition* as "a generalized state associated with a significantly increased risk of oral cancer". The former lesions include leukoplakia and erythroplakia. The latter conditions include syphilis, sideropenic dysphagia (Plummer–Vinson syndrome), submucous fibrosis, lichen planus, discoid lupus erythematosus and actinic keratosis, all of which are associated with mucosal atrophy and altered mucosal homeostasis without a discrete lesion being visible clinically.

Leukoplakia, a white patch which by exclusion is not any other disease, has been shown in one large study in Sweden [2] to be present in 3%–4% of people aged over 40 years, thus being much more common than the cumulative incidence of oral cancer. The evidence that some leukoplakias and erythroplakias (red patches) are precancerous comes from studies showing that these lesions are sometimes associated with oral cancers, and a few longitudinal studies, in which leukoplakias have subsequently developed malignant change [82]. The cases of leukoplakia in the latter are generally those seen in hospital series and cannot be assumed to be typical of all leukoplakias in the population. The most important determinant of risk of progression is the presence of epithelial dysplasia on histological examination, which may be present in 15%–54% of cases of leukoplakia [66] and 85% of cases of erythroplakia [78]. One follow-up study over 8 years in the USA found that 20% of leukoplakias became malignant, 20% progressed to more severe dysplasia, 20% regressed and the remaining 40% showed no change [53]. A similar 10 year follow-up in India [32] found that 10% became malignant, 30% increased in severity, and 13% regressed. Factors influencing the likelihood of progression are the severity of dysplasia, the colour (red or speckled red lesions having higher risk), the texture (nodular lesions being at greater risk than smooth) and the site within the oral cavity (floor of the mouth and lateral border of the tongue being at higher risk) [82]. Laboratory research into markers of malignant potential, such as ploidy and genetic mutations, have mainly concentrated on invasive cancers rather than precancerous lesions, and have implicated various members of the *ras* family of oncogenes, and *p53*. In a comprehensive review of cellular and molecular markers of risk in oral precancerous lesions and conditions, Johnson et al. [42] conclude that rapid progress will soon be made in understanding the series of genetic events leading to malignant transformation of oropharyngeal epithelia. But in the meantime reliance will still have to be placed on clinical and histological features.

It is claimed that the majority of oral cancers are preceded by a clinically detectable lesion [67] but the proportion which do *not* go through such a stage is not precisely known.

Prognosis of Invasive Oral Cancer

The 5-year relative survival for patients in the UK with cancers of the tongue, gum and floor of mouth diagnosed in 1981 was around 40% for men and 50% for women but cancers of the lip have a much better prognosis (94% for men, 71% for women) [18]. There has been little recent improvement in overall survival but, as with other cancers, survival is strongly dependent on size, depth of infiltration and involvement of lymph nodes. Extrapolating from one large German study [69], Speight et al. [82] estimate a 5-year survival of 72% for lesions of less than 4 cm diameter or less than 5 mm depth of invasion, falling to 46% for lesions with a diameter greater than 4 cm and depth of invasion greater than 5 mm.

Rationale for Screening

Screening could be used to detect both precancerous lesions and early invasive cancers. The intervention which can be offered for the latter group is surgical excision, which if the cancer is small and without lymphatic spread, can be done with minimal disfigurement and without the necessity for radiotherapy. For precancerous lesions the intervention depends on assessment of the risk of progression – ideally by histological assessment of dysplasia in a biopsy specimen. Low-risk lesions can be managed by surveillance at regular intervals, whereas high-risk lesions can be excised surgically or by cryosurgery or laser. Some clinicians also advocate topical chemotherapy and systemic retinoid treatment [46].

For all patients identified by screening, the opportunity can be taken to assess their personal risk of further oral cancer or precancer, and, where relevant, to encourage them to cut down on tobacco and alcohol. At least one study [11] has demonstrated that oral mucosa became less dysplastic following cessation of smoking.

The Screening Test

Visual examination of the mouth using oral mirrors is the primary screening method. In populations where regular dental examination is common, it is assumed that dentists in the course of their daily work undertake oral neoplasia screening; in this context screening is often referred to as opportunistic screening or "case-finding". In other populations it may be necessary to set up a formal organised system of screening in order to obtain reasonable coverage of the population.

Visual examination is not suitable for detection of most pharyngeal lesions, therefore its sensitivity is judged on its ability to detect neoplasia in the lip, tongue, floor of mouth, gum, and buccal mucosa.

The sensitivity and specificity of clinical examination has not yet been adequately studied in a screening context. False negative results of dental and medical examinations of the mouth in symptomatic patients have been noted in some early studies [21, 70, 79]. This suggests that both dentists and general practitioners may require specific education in oral cancer and precancer detection, if opportunistic case-finding is to work [78].

Education of primary health workers in Sri Lanka has shown that they can be trained to recognise both precancerous lesions and early cancers [94]. Among people they referred and who attended for specialist assessment, the diagnosis was correct in 89%. However, in this study only 54% of those referred actually attended, so it is not possible to derive estimates of specificity and predictive value, and since there was no follow-up sensitivity is also unknown.

Studies have now been started in the UK to assess the sensitivity, specificity and positive predictive value of screening by dental practitioners.

Compliance

Lack of acceptability of oral examination is likely to prove a major obstacle to evaluation of oral cancer screening. In the UK only 50% of the population regularly attend a dentist [87], and attendance is lower in the elderly and in unskilled social classes among whom smoking is more prevalent. Thus opportunistic screening by dentists will only reach a minority of those at risk of oral cancer. Opportunistic screening by general medical practitioners would be more likely to include high risk groups, but would require a major educational programme for general practitioners to acquire the necessary skill and commitment to undertake oral cancer screening. Screening by invitation from a population register has been shown to achieve reasonably high compliance for other cancer sites. However, one study in London found that only 25% of 3826 men and women aged over 40 years accepted an invitation for oral cancer screening by dental practitioners in their general medical practitioner's health centre; the inclusion of an information leaflet made no difference to response (Jullien, personal communication).

In the developing world, screening can, in theory, be implemented by systematically recruiting all subjects of the relevant age-group in rural villages, workplaces, etc., or, as in the Sri Lanka study [93], by opportunistic screening of people consulting health workers about other conditions. A problem, particularly with the latter approach, is that subjects may agree to be examined without understanding its purpose, nor the implications of being found positive and this may lead to poor compliance with attendance for investigation of possible lesions.

The Benefits of Screening

As yet, no study has demonstrated a reduced incidence of oral cancer resulting from screening for preneoplasia, nor reduced mortality resulting from screening for early cancer. There have been no randomised trials of screening programmes, nor any retrospective evaluations. Thus the benefits of screening for oral cancer are still completely unproven.

The Costs of Screening

Likewise the costs and disadvantages of screening have not yet been quantified. It seems likely that one of the most important disadvantages, both in causing unnecessary morbidity and in its use of resources, will arise from the treatment and surveillance of many cases of leukoplakia, the majority of which would not in any case progress to malignancy.

Conclusions

Screening for oral cancer, although opportunistically practised to an unknown extent and with variable quality, is at an early point in evaluation. Further research is required into issues relevant to its benefit (sensitivity, acceptability, compliance with referral) and its cost (specificity, natural history of leukoplakia). Ideally such research should be built into large randomised controlled trials designed to demonstrate whether, and by how much, screening can reduce incidence and mortality, and to quantify its morbidity and resource costs. Until the results of such trials are available, it is premature to introduce further oral cancer screening, other than in a research context.

References

1. Auerbach O, Hammond EC, Garfinkel L (1979) Changes in bronchial epithelium in relation to cigarette smoking, 1955–1960 vs 1970–1977. N Engl J Med 300:381–386.
2. Axell T (1987) Occurrence of leukoplakia and some other oral white lesions among 20 333 adult Swedish people. Community Dent Oral Epidemiol 15:46–51.
3. Bailar JC (1984) Screening for lung cancer – where are we now? Am Rev Respir Dis 130:541–542.
4. Barker DJ, Coggon D, Holdsmond C, Wickham C (1990) Poor housing and high rates of stomach cancer in England and Wales. Br J Cancer 61:575–578.
5. Beckwith JB, Perrin EV (1963) In-situ neuroblastomas: a contribution to the natural history of neural crest tumours. Am J Pathol 43:1089–1104.
6. Berlin NI, Buncher CR, Fontana RS, Frost JK, Melamed MR (1984) The National Cancer Institute Cooperative Early Lung Cancer Detection Program. Results of the initial screen (prevalence). Early lung cancer detection: introduction. Am Rev Respir Dis 130:545–549.
7. Bernstein ML, Leclerc JM, Bunin G et al. (1992) A population-based study of neuroblastoma incidence, survival and mortality in North America. J Clin Oncol 10:323–329.
8. Besscho F, Hashizuma K, Nakajo T, Kamoshita S (1991) Mass screening in Japan increased the detection of infants with neuroblastoma without a decrease in cases in older children. J Pediatr 119:237–241.
9. Birrer MJ, Brown PH (1992) Application of molecular genetics to the early diagnosis and screening of lung cancer. Cancer Res (Suppl) 52:2658–2664.
10. Black RJ, Sharp L, Kendrick SW (1993) Trends in cancer survival in Scotland 1968–1990. ISD Publications, Edinburgh.
11. Blot WJ, McLaughlin JK, Wynn DM et al. (1988) Smoking and drinking in relation to oral and pharyngeal cancer. Cancer Res 48:3282–3287.

12. Blot WJ (1992) Alcohol and cancer. Cancer Res 50(Suppl):2119–2123.
13. Boyle P, Macfarlane GJ, Maisonneuve P, Zheng T (1990) Epidemiology of mouth cancer in 1989: a review. J R Soc Med 83:724–730.
14. Boyle P, Macfarlane GJ, Scully C (1993) Oral cancer: necessity for prevention strategies. Lancet 342:1129.
15. Brett GZ (1968) The value of lung cancer detection by six-monthly chest radiographs. Thorax 23:414–420.
16. Brodeur GM, Hayes FA, Green AA et al. (1987) Consistent N-myc copy number in simultaneous or consecutive neuroblastoma samples from sixty individual patients. Cancer Res 47:4248–4253.
17. Brodeur GM, Pritchard J, Berthold F et al. (1993) Revisions of the International Criteria for Neuroblastoma Diagnosis, Staging and Response to Treatment. J Clin Oncol 11:1466–1477.
18. Cancer Research Campaign (1990) Fact Sheet 14: Oral Cancer.
19. Cancer Research Campaign (1992) Fact Sheet 11: Lung Cancer.
20. Chamberlain J (1994) Screening for neuroblastoma. A review of the evidence. J Med Screening 1:169–175.
21. Coffin F (1964) Cancer and the dental surgeon. Br Dental J 116:191–202.
22. Coldman AJ, Fryer CH, Elwood JM, Sonley MJ (1980) Neuroblastoma: influence of age at diagnosis, stage, tumour site and sex on prognosis. Cancer 46:1896–1901.
23. Doll R, Peto R (1976) Mortality in relation to smoking: 20 years' observation on British male doctors. Br Med J iv:1525–1526.
24. Draper GJ, Birch JM, Bithell JF et al. (1982) Childhood cancer in Britain. Studies on medical and population subjects, No. 37. HMSO, London.
25. Ebeling K, Nischan P (1987) Screening for lung cancer – results from a case-control study. Int J Cancer 40:141–144.
26. Eddy DM (1989) Screening for lung cancer. Ann Intern Med 111:232–237.
27. Eurogast Study Group (1993) An international association between *Helicobacter pylori* infection and gastric cancer. Lancet 341:1359–1362.
28. Flehinger BJ, Melamed Mr, Zaman MB et al. (1984) Screening for early detection of lung cancer in New York. In: Prorok PC, Miller AB (eds) Screening for cancer. I. General principles on evaluation of screening for cancer and screening for lung, bladder and oral cancer. UICC Technical Report Series, 78, Geneva, pp 123–135.
29. Fontana RS, Sanderson DR, Woolner LB, Taylor WF, Miller WE, Muhm JR (1986) Lung cancer screening: The Mayo Program. J Occup Med 28:746–750.
30. Fukao A, Hisamichi S, Sugawara N (1987) A case-control study on evaluating the effect of mass screening on decreasing advanced stomach cancer. J Jpn Soc Gastroenterol Mass Surv 75:112–116.
31. Goodwin CS (1993) Gastric cancer and *Helicobacter pylori:* the whispering killer? Lancet 342:507–508.
32. Gupta PC, Mehta FS, Daftary DK et al. (1980) Incidence rates of oral cancers and natural history of oral precancerous lesions in a 10 year follow up study of Indian villages. Community Dental Oral Epidemiol 8:287–333.
33. Hakama M, Pukkala E (1988) Evaluation of an immunological screening for stomach cancer. In: Chamberlain J, Miller AB (eds) Screening for gastrointestinal cancer. International Union Against Cancer. Hans Huber, Toronto, pp 71–75.
34. Hakama M, Stenman U-H, Knekt P et al. (1994) Tumour markers and screening for gastrointestinal cancer: a follow up study in Finland. J Med Screening 1:60–64.
35. Hallissey MT, Allum WH, Jewkes AJ, Ellis DJ, Fielding JWL (1990) Early detection of

gastric cancer. Br Med J 301:513–515.

36. Hanawa Y, Sawada T, Tsunoda A (1990) Decrease in childhood neuroblastoma death in Japan. Med Pediatr Oncol 18:472–475.

37. Hayashi Y, Kanda N, Inaba T et al. (1989) Cytogenetic findings and prognosis in neuroblastoma with emphasis on marker chromosome 1. Cancer 63:126–132.

38. Hisamichi A, Fukao A, Sugawara N et al. (1991) Evaluation of mass screening programme for stomach cancer in Japan. In: Miller AB, Chamberlain J, Day NE, Hakama M, Prorok PC (eds) Cancer Screening. International Union Against Cancer. Cambridge University Press, Cambridge, pp 357–370.

39. International Agency for Research on Cancer (1985) Tobacco habits other than smoking, betel quid and areca-nut chewing; and some related nitrosamines. IARC Monographs on the evaluation of carcinogenic risk of chemicals to humans. IARC 37, Lyon.

40. International Agency for Research on Cancer (1989) Monograph 42: alcoholic beverages. IARC, Lyon.

41. Ishimoto K, Kiyokawa N, Fujita H et al. (1990) Problems of mass screening for neuroblastoma = analysis of false negative cases. J Pediatr Surg 5:398–401.

42. Johnson NW, Ranasinghe AW, Warnakulasuriya KAAS (1993) Potentially malignant lesions and conditions of the mouth and oropharynx: natural history – cellular and molecular markers of risk. Eur J Cancer 2(2):31–51.

43. Kaneko Y, Kanda N, Maseki N et al. (1990) Current urinary mass screening for catecholamine metabolities at 6 months of age may be detecting only a small portion of high-risk neuroblastomas: a chromosome and N-myc amplification study. J Clin Oncol 8:2005–2013.

44. Knudson AG, Meadow AT (1980) Regression of neuroblastoma IVS: a genetic hypothesis. N Engl J Med 302:1254–1256.

45. Kubik A, Parkin DM, Khlat M, Erban J, Polak J, Adamec M (1990) Lack of benefit from semi-annual screening for cancer of the lung: follow-up report of a randomized controlled trial on a population of high-risk males in Czechoslovakia. Int J Cancer 45:26–33.

46. Lamay P-J (1993) Management options in potentially malignant and malignant oral epithelial lesions. Community Dental Health 10(1):53–62.

47. Lancet (1986) Oral snuff: a preventable carcinogenic hazard. Lancet i:198–201.

48. McLoughlin JK, Gridley G, Block G et al. (1988) Dietary factors in oral and pharyngeal cancer. J Natl Cancer Inst 80:1237–1243.

49. Malaowalla AM, Silverman S, Mani NJ, Bilimoria KF, Smith LW (1976) Oral cancer in 57518 industrial workers in Gujarat, India. Cancer 37:1882–1886.

50. Matsumara M, Tsunoda A, Nishi T, Nishihira H, Sasaki Y (1991) Spontaneous regression of neuroblastoma detected by mass screening. Lancet 338:447–448.

51. Melamed MR, Flehinger BJ, Zaman MB et al. (1984) Screening for lung cancer. Results of the Memorial Sloan–Kettering study in New York. Chest 86:44–53.

52. Miller AB (1989) Vitamins, minerals and other dietary factors. In: Miller AB (ed) Diet and the aetiology of cancer. Springer-Verlag, Berlin, pp 39–54.

53. Mincer HH, Coleman SA, Hopkins KP (1972) Observations on the clinical characteristics of oral lesions showing histologic epithelial dysplasia. Oral Surg Oral Med Oral Pathol 33:389–399.

54. Morson BC (1955) Intestinal metaplasia of gastric mucosa. Br J Cancer 9:365–376.

55. Naito H, Sasaki M, Yamashiro K et al. (1990) Improvement in prognosis of neuroblastoma through mass population screening. J Pediatr Surg 25:245–248.

56. Nash FA, Morgan JM, Tomkins JG (1968) South London lung cancer study. Br Med J 2:715–721.
57. Nishi M, Miyake H, Takeda T et al. (1987) Effects of the mass screening of neuroblastoma in Sapporo City. Cancer 60:433–435.
58. Nishi M, Miyake H, Takeda T, Takasugi N, Hanai J, Kawai T (1991) Mass screening for neuroblastoma and estimation of costs. Acta Paediatr Scand 80:812–817.
59. Office of Population Censuses and Surveys (1993) Cancer statistics. Registrations. Series MB1 no. 20. HMSO, London.
60. Office of Population Censuses and Surveys (1993) Mortality statistics. Cause. Series DH2 no. 19. HMSO, London.
61. Oshima A, Hirata N, Ubukata T, Umeda K, Fujimoto I (1986) Evaluation of a mass screening program for stomach cancer with a case-control study design. Int J Cancer 38:829–833.
62. Parker L, Craft AW, Dale G et al. (1992) Screening for neuroblastoma in the North of England. Br Med J 305:1260–1263.
63. Parkin DM, Laara E, Muir CS (1988) Estimates of the worldwide frequency of sixteen major cancers in 1980. Int J Cancer 41:184–197.
64. Parkin DM, Stiller CA, Draper GJ et al. (1988) International incidence of childhood cancer. IARC, Scientific Publications, No. 87, Lyon, 1988.
65. Peto R (1994) Smoking and death: the past 40 years and the next 40. Br Med J 309:937–939.
66. Pindborg JJ (1980) Oral cancer and precancer. John Wright and Sons Ltd, Bristol.
67. Pindborg JJ, Daftary DK, Gupta P et al. (1991) Public health aspects of oral cancer: implications for cancer prevention in the community. In: Johnson NW (ed) Risk markers for oral cancer: detection of patients and lesions at risk, Vol 2. Cambridge University Press, Cambridge, pp 380–388.
68. Pisani P, Oliver WE, Parkin DM, Alvarez N (1994) Case-control study of gastric cancer screening in Venezuela. Br J Cancer 69:1102–1105.
69. Platz H, Fries R, Hudec M (1986) Prognoses of oral cavity carcinomas. Carl Hanser Verlag, Munich, pp 187.
70. Pogrel MA (1974) The dentist and oral cancer in the north east of Scotland. Br Dental J 137:15–20.
71. Prorok PC, Byar DP, Smart CR, Baker SG, Connor RJ (1991) Evaluation of screening for prostate, lung and colorectal cancers: the PLC trial. In: Miller AB, Chamberlain J, Day NE, Hakama M, Prorok PC (eds) Cancer screening. Cambridge University Press, Cambridge, pp 300–321.
72. Saccomano G, Archer VE, Auerbach O, Saunders RP, Brennan LM (1974) Development of carcinoma of the lung as reflected in exfoliated cells. Cancer 33:256–270.
73. Sankila R, Hakama M (1993) Survival trends for neuroblastoma in Finland: negative reflections on screening. Eur J Cancer 29:122–123.
74. Sawada T, Kidowaki T, Sakamoto I et al. (1984) Neuroblastoma: mass screening for early detection and its prognosis. Cancer 53:2731–2735.
75. Sawada T, Kawakatu H, Sugimoto T (1987) Screening for neuroblastoma. Lancet ii:1204.
76. Sawada T, Matsumara T, Matsuda Y, Kawakatsu H (1991) Neuroblastoma studies in Japan. In: Miller AB, Chamberlain J, Day NE, Hakama M, Prorok PC (eds) Cancer screening. Cambridge University Press, Cambridge, pp 325–336.
77. Schnetler JFC (1992) Oral cancer diagnosis and delays in referral. Br J Oral Maxillofacial Surg 30:210–213.

78. Scully C (1993) Clinical diagnostic methods for the detection of premalignant and early malignant oral lesions. Community Dental Health 10(1):43–52.
79. Shafer WG (1975) Initial mismanagement and delay in diagnosis of oral cancers. J Am Dent Assoc 90: 1262–1264.
80. Sobue T, Suzuki T, Naruke T and The Japanese Lung Cancer Screening Research Group (1992) A case-control study for evaluating lung cancer screening in Japan. Int J Cancer 50:230–237.
81. Souhami R (1992) Lung cancer. Br Med J 304:1298–1301.
82. Speight PM, Morgan PR (1993) The natural history and pathology of oral cancer and precancer. Community Dental Health 10(1):31–41.
83. Stiller CA, Bunch KJ (1990) Trends in survival for childhood cancer diagnosed 1971–85. Br J Cancer 62:806–816.
84. Stiller CA (1993) Trends in neuroblastoma in Great Britain: incidence and mortality, 1971–1990. Eur J Cancer 29A:1008–1012.
85. Sue-Ling HM, Johnston D, Martin IC et al. (1993) Gastric cancer: a curable disease in Britain. Br Med J 307:591–596.
86. Tockman MS, Frost JK, Stitik FP et al. (1985) Screening and detection of lung cancer. In: Aisner J (ed) Lung cancer. Churchill Livingstone, New York, pp 25–29.
87. Todd J, Lader D (1991) Adult dental health, United Kingdom 1988. HMSO, London.
88. Tsukuma T, Mishima T, Oshima A (1983) Prospective study of "early" gastric cancer. Int J Cancer 31:421–426.
89. Tuchman M, Lemieux B, Auray-Blais C et al. (1990) Screening for neuroblastoma at three weeks of age: methods and preliminary results from the Quebec neuroblastoma screening project. Pediatrics 86:765–773.
90. Tuchman M, Ramnaraine ML, Woods WG et al. (1987) Three years of experience with random urinary homovanillic and vanillylmandelic acid levels in the diagnosis of neuroblastoma. Pediatrics 79:203–205.
91. Walter SD, Kubik A, Parkin DM, Reissigova J, Adamec M, Khlat M (1992) The natural history of lung cancer estimated from the results of a randomized trial of screening. Cancer Causes and Control 3:115–123.
92. Wang B, Yanagawa H, Sakata K (1994) Gastric cancer screening programme in Japan: how to improve its implementation in the community. J Epidemiol Community Health 48:182–187.
93. Warnakulasuriya S, Ekanayake A, Stjernsward J, Pindborg JJ, Sivayoham S (1988) Compliance following referral in the early detection of oral cancer and precancer in Sri Lanka. Community Dent Oral Epidemiol 16:326–329.
94. Warnakulasuriya S, Pindborg JJ (1990) Reliability of oral precancer screening by primary health care workers in Sri Lanka. Comm Dental Hlth 7:73–79.
95. Weiss W (1984) Implications of tumor growth rate for the natural history of lung cancer. J Occup Med 26:345–352
96. Woods WG, Lemieux B, Tuchman M (1992) Neuroblastoma represents distinct clinical–biological entities: a review and perspective from the Quebec neuroblastoma screening project. Pediatrics 89:114–118.
97. World Health Organization (1978) Definitions of leukoplakia and related lesions: an aid to studies on oral precancer. Oral Surg Oral Med Oral Pathol 46:518–539.

9 – Psychological Aspects of Cancer Screening

Ruth Ellman

Introduction

This chapter considers the effect of cancer screening on psychological morbidity and the importance of psychological factors to the success of screening programmes. There is ample evidence that patients with newly diagnosed or recurrent cancer suffer psychological morbidity, some of which is avoidable. Physical symptoms of the disease, effects of different treatments and apprehensions about metastasis and death cause some inevitable distress but additional distress is often caused unnecessarily by the patient's misconceptions and by suboptimal care. Interest in measuring the distress caused specifically by screening is recent, arising from the contention that a cancer screening test, although capable of reducing mortality, might yet not be justified if the psychological harm associated with screening outweighed the benefit [43, 56].

Research Methodology

It is important to distinguish distress which is due to cancer screening from distress which is due to the cancer itself or to unrelated factors. Rigorous and self critical qualitative research indicates the types of problems which arise with screening but quantitative research in this area is particularly difficult. Three ways in which screening may lead to psychological morbidity have been postulated. Firstly, the process of being encouraged to accept screening may increase anxiety by raising awareness about vulnerability to the cancer concerned. Secondly, anxiety is inevitably caused when an asymptomatic person has a positive screening test, and, for those which turn out to be false positives, this may be a serious unwanted side-effect of the screening programme. Thirdly, in patients with screen-detected cancer, anxiety may be greater than in other cancer patients because of their previous asymptomatic state. Different research methods are applicable for studying these three potential sources of psychological morbidity, but all must observe general epidemiological rules and must include a valid comparison or control group.

For a study of the psychological effects of encouraging screening, comparing individuals randomised into screening and control groups is not ideal as the randomisation, rather than the screening, can arouse anxiety among those singled out from their neighbours and may also lead to poor compliance. Cluster random-isation may be better but the organisation of sufficiently large studies on such a basis is daunting and no studies of the psychological effects of screening have had such controls. For a study of the effect on well-being of false positive screening reports, screened subjects with normal results can serve as a comparison group. However, it should be kept in mind that abnormalities giving rise to the false positive results may have worried the patient before attending and may have affected the decision to come. For a study of the effect on cancer patients of screen detection it may be difficult to find a suitable comparison group once mass screen-ing is on general offer since those who have detected lesions by chance self-exam-ination are likely to have been influenced by the screening programme in one way or another: they may have regrets if they were not invited, be angry if they were passed as normal or feel guilty if they refused their invitation.

The size of study should be adequate to ensure that there is a high probability that a difference of clinical importance is detectable and that a negative result will carry some weight; small studies lead to publication bias in favour of studies which chance to yield positive findings.

Psychological studies are easily distorted by selection bias; agreement to answer questions is affected by feelings of dependence or gratefulness towards staff, by beliefs about whether psychological morbidity is an important aspect of health and by whether a subject is seeking to cope with distress by denying its existence. Likewise psychological studies are particularly susceptible to recall bias; recall of a previous state of mind is likely to be influenced by current feelings and, unlike recall of objective events, a previous state of mind cannot be externally verified.

Prospective studies overcome some of the problems but the timing of question-ing presents difficulties. Since questioning cannot start before patients present at a clinic the cumulative distress experienced by symptomatic patients may be under-estimated when comparing them with patients whose abnormality is first noticed at screening. Frequent questioning may alter the type of answer given yet without frequent questioning peaks of distress may be missed and lead to underestimation of cumulative distress. Dwindling response rates make it difficult to assess the longer term results; very few studies have attempted to follow patients for more than a year.

The usefulness of a number of different questionnaires for assessing quality of life in cancer patients has been reviewed by Maguire and Selby [32]. For psychiatric morbidity they considered the General Health Questionnaire (GHQ), the Hospital Anxiety and Depression (HAD) scale and the Rotterdam Checklist (RCL) both acceptable and valid in cancer patients. The validity of the latter two has not been fully tested for use in people without physical illness. In aiming at brevity and acceptability these questionnaires are obliged to leave out some common aspects of morbidity.

The choice of a threshold score for the definition of a probable case of anxiety or depression with these questionnaires depends on whether the primary aim is to identify subjects with clinically significant morbidity, to estimate prevalence within a single population or to detect significant differences between groups. For clinical psychiatric purposes the cut-off can be set to provide optimal agreement with local assessment by an interviewer or adjusted according to whether positive or negative misclassification is considered worse. For a best estimate of prevalence the threshold should be chosen to minimise bias, a higher threshold being adopted where prevalence is low. For comparing morbidity in two groups the cut-off point must be the same in the two groups and the comparison of the distribution of test scores rather than simply the prevalence of "cases" provides a more sensitive measure of difference.

Administration of questionnaires by trained interviewers, rather than by self-completion, enables other cues besides direct answers to questions to be taken into account and is more successful at identifying patients who would benefit from treatment, but introduces an added source of bias in comparative studies.

In all of these types of questionnaire subjects are expected to compare their feelings with a supposed norm or with their "usual" state. The threshold for commenting on a symptom may be altered if the subject is used to it, has previously experienced it in a more extreme form or thinks it is only to be expected in the circumstances. Some questionnaires ask about emotions attributed to cancer or screening [4] whereas others are not intended to be context specific. In practice, distress may well be multifactorial, the cause difficult to tell, and the subject tempted to blame emotions of unknown origin on the suggested event.

Trade-off methods provide an alternative way of assessing the severity of distress, and are favoured by economists. Subjects – sometimes patients, sometimes medical experts and sometimes representatives of the public – are asked what they would be willing to pay to obtain or avoid an experience [14] or, even more hypothetically, the number of days of life they would be willing to trade-off to avoid some adverse experience [48]. Medical experts and members of the public tend to value the quality of life with cancer lower than patients themselves [45]. It is arguable whose evaluation is the more relevant for economic studies.

The limitations of research methods should be borne in mind when considering the literature which is reviewed below.

Psychological Effects of Invitation to Screening

Those who have least cause for distress are those who are simply invited to screening and are passed as normal. Complaints of distress resulting simply from receiving an invitation are reported [6, 37] but their importance is probably small. Dean et al. [6] compared psychological morbidity in 132 women screened for breast cancer and found negative three months previously with morbidity reported by a population sample randomly selected before screening invitations were sent out. Of the screened women 30% said that they had been made anxious by the invitation and 20% by the actual screening. About 8% felt that the procedure had had the lasting effect of making them more anxious about breast cancer. Despite this there was no evidence from their responses to the GHQ that they were more anxious or depressed than the population sample. Another study of the effects of breast cancer screening [8] included a group of screen-normal women whose scores for anxiety were significantly lower at three months than they had been when they filled the questionnaire in at a clinic. The women's initial scores may have been raised above their usual level due to screening or perhaps their later scores were lowered due to a beneficial effect of reassurance. Possibly women become less anxious about breast cancer after screening or, if initially scared that the medical encounter will be unnerving gain some general self-confidence from finding that it is tolerable. In Norway, Gram and Slenker [15] concluded that there was a beneficial effect when they found a lower prevalence of anxiety among screen-negative women six months after screening than among women from a nearby city who had not been offered screening. In Australia, Cockburn et al. [4] found no significant differences between routinely screened women and randomly selected controls from neighbouring regions. If increasing medicalisation really adds to the stress of life its effect may well be too subtle to be detected by a short questionnaire.

Psychological Effects of a Positive Screening Test

One of the main drawbacks of screening is the possibility of recall for an abnormality which will ultimately prove benign. The distress occasioned by recall can be severe as anyone working in recall clinics will be aware. It has been most thoroughly studied in breast cancer screening. Five such studies [2, 4, 8, 14, 25] which have examined the effect of recall following mammographic screening in response to invitation are summarised in Table 9.1 and several more studies are in progress [38]. In each of the published studies women with false positive screening results were compared with women with negative screening test results. All the studies agree that distress is increased by recall but four of them suggest that, although anxiety may still be raised a week after reassurance, 3–18 months afterwards it is back to normal or similar to that of the screen-negative group. Gram et al. [14, 15] found that women were still anxious about breast cancer 6 months after reassurance but that such anxiety was strongly related to anxiety reported to have been present before screening. Only Lerman et al.'s [25] study found that women with false positive screening reported that concerns about breast cancer were still disturbing their emotional and physical well-being three months after screening. This might be because of differences in the study method or in the way that screening in this American programme was organised – 20% were advised to seek follow-up through their general physicians and a considerable proportion, including some with high suspicion of cancer, did not have further investigations whereas in the European studies follow-up investigation was an integral part of the screening service. Surgical biopsy may also have been more common, as it was generally in the USA at this time, but was not reported separately from needle aspiration. Gram et al. [14] found that 33% of those who had had biopsy had persistent pain or dysthesia at 6 months and 5/30 of them remembered their experience as the worst thing that had ever happened to them.

In screening for cervical cancer the distinction between false positive and true positive screening results is not as clear cut as in breast cancer screening. Whereas the great majority of breast cancers picked up by screening are invasive, the aim of cervical screening is to pick up all cases at a preinvasive stage. It is probable, on epidemiological evidence [52], that a considerable proportion would never progress to symptomatic cancer if left undiscovered, yet, since treatment can now often be given as a minor outpatient procedure, the threshold for calling a case positive and recommending treatment has been lowered. Women recalled after cervical screening have a very low probability of dying of cervical cancer, even if they ignore advice – much lower than the probability for recalled breast screening patients, of dying of breast cancer.

Table 9.1   Studies of psychological morbidity among women recalled after mammography

Study	Group and size		Questionnaire	Findings in false positive group
Ellman et al. [8] UK	Scr-ve	302	GHQ (general) plus interview on consumer opinion	Distress high at recall but not at 3 months
	False+ve	300		
	Symptoms	150		
Gram et al. [14] Norway	Scr-ve	126	Self-anchoring scale (general) plus Q's re Br Cancer plus interview on cost relative to other stresses	Distress during follow-up but not at 18 months though still anxious about breast cancer
	False+ve	152		
Lerman et al. [25] USA	Scr-ve	121	Q's re Br Cancer; telephone interview	Mood and function still disturbed by thoughts about breast cancer 3 months after screening
	False+ve	187		
Bull and Campbell [2] UK	Scr-ve	420	HAD (general) plus Q on effect of screening on anxiety	Distress not increased at 6 weeks even among those biopsied
	False+ve (non-biopsied)	240		
	False+ve (biopsied)	68		
Cockburn et al. [4] Australia	Scr-ve	142	Q's re Br Cancer; telephone interview	Distress at 1 week after reassurance but not at 8 months
	False+ve (non-biopsied)	58		
	Unscr pop	52		

As with breast cancer screening, high levels of distress are found in women awaiting investigation of abnormal smear results. Levels of anxiety comparable to those of patients awaiting major surgery have been reported [22, 34, 54]. This is particularly serious where women have to wait several months for colposcopy. Kincey et al. [22] noted that the women were poorly informed about colposcopy and dissatisfied with the information they had been given, suggesting that some anxiety might be avoidable by better communication. Wilkinson et al. [54] confirmed, in a small randomised trial, that leaflets sent out with a recall letter reduce anxiety in those awaiting investigation of an abnormal smear. Anxiety may lead to refusal of follow-up [25]. There is also evidence that distress sometimes persists after full investigation and/or treatment. Posner and Vessey [41], in a detailed qualitative study of 153 women who had been referred for colposcopic investigation, found that 65% reported distress on receiving the letter recommending further investigation, that 35% still felt at risk of cancer after treatment and that 52% of them reported feelings of self-disgust or altered attitudes to their sexual relationships. Reelick et al. [42], in a study comparing women with positive and negative results, found significant differences in reported ill-health, gloominess and nervousness one week after receiving smear test results but after full investigation and treatment it was only among those who had been admitted to hospital for operative treatment that persistent psychological or somatic problems were reported. Distress was related to concerns expressed before treatment about menstruation and fertility which may indeed be adversely affected by treatment for CIN [28]. Persistent disturbance was also reported by Campion et al. [3]: six months after diagnosis and treatment at a colposcopy clinic, women with CIN were significantly more likely to have psychosexual problems than women being investigated for sexually transmitted disease who did not have CIN.

A few small studies of psychological responses have been included in screening programmes which are still of unproven value. In screening for colorectal cancer Mant et al. [33] found that three out of 54 people with false positive faecal occult blood tests were still anxious following reassurance that further investigations were all negative. Brandberg et al. [1], in a study conducted 7 months after screening for melanoma, found no difference in HAD scores or psychosomatic complaints between 37 people who had had suspicious moles excised and the large majority who had had no suspicious lesions.

More surprisingly little distress attributable to screening for ovarian cancer was found in 302 women attending because of high familial risk [53]. They were anxious before attending screening but, despite the fact that 69 had false positive results and 20 of them underwent hysterectomy and bilateral oophorectomy, GHQ scores returned to their prescreening values by 3 months even among those who underwent surgery. The authors point out that this was a study of highly self-selected women and may not reflect how low-risk women invited to mass screening would behave. Women with higher than average levels of anxiety are over-represented both among those who make special efforts to get screened and among those who avoid it. They may, therefore, be over-represented in groups who have taken the initiative to seek investigation. In a study which included symptomatic women who had been referred for investigation [8], distress was still increased at 3 months despite reassurance that breast cancer was not the cause of the symptoms. This was in contrast to the women who had false positive results from screening, among whom distress was only temporary. Underlying psychological morbidity, not likely to be resolved by referral to a surgeon, may, in some cases, have expressed itself in concern about a breast problem and so led to referral.

The introduction of widespread genetic screening for cancer would introduce new psychosocial problems [11] perhaps similar to, but less extreme than, those which have been documented in screening for Huntington's Chorea [47], because the cancers would be assumed to be preventable.

Psychological Effects in Patients with Screen-Detected Cancer

It is against a background of cancer-induced psychological morbidity and considerable variation in treatment that assesment is needed of whether cancer patients whose cancer was detected by screening suffer any more or less distress than they would have done had screening not been provided. Table 9.2 (opposite) shows the phases experienced by the patient in the absence of screening. Screening will bring forward Phases 2 and 3 to an earlier age. This is a possible disadvantage since, in general, the distress caused by illness at a younger age may be greater, both for the subject and dependants. A phase during which invitation, screening and waiting for recall occur will be substituted for Phase 1. It is difficult to discover which of these is worse since patients may be questioned about their feelings during the screening-to-recall phase but cannot be questioned, except retrospectively, about feelings while uncertain whether to seek medical investigation; some patients delay for many months. In Phases 2 and 3 the screen-detected patient should theoretically benefit from having a smaller, less advanced cancer with a more favourable prognosis which can be satisfactorily treated by less aggressive methods. On the other hand it has been suggested [31] that screen-detected cancer patients might suffer more, because of different attitudes to the cancer. They might be uncertain about whether the symptomless cancer was real, more anxious that recurrence might develop insidiously, have less time to adjust to the realisation that treatment was necessary and perhaps experience anger that it was not picked up by screening at a preinvasive stage. Phase 4 will be prolonged by screening both because of the shift in age at diagnosis and because for some patients screening truly prolongs life. Fewer screen-detected patients will ever experience Phase 5.

Table 9.2   Phases of potential distress in symptomatic cancer patients

Phase 0	Background distress, unaware of cancer
Phase 1	Distress while uncertain whether symptoms merit self-referral
Phase 2	Distress while under investigation
Phase 3	Distress during treatment, and while adjusting to changed state
Phase 4	Distress in stable, disease free state
Phase 5	Distress of recurrence and terminal illness

There is, in fact, little evidence that, among operable symptom-presenting cancers, stage differences determine the level of distress experienced. This may be because, though doctors no longer hide the diagnosis of cancer from the patient, patients are encouraged to believe that their disease has been adequately dealt with. Only the patient who has special knowledge or is persistent in questioning is likely to learn if the prognosis is worse than average. Nor is the treatment for early disease necessarily less unpleasant than that for advanced disease. In breast cancer radical mastectomy is no longer a recommended form of treatment but simple mastectomy may be used for early stage or even non-invasive breast cancer and adjuvant chemotherapy may be used for early invasive breast cancer whereas patients with advanced disease may be treated with the far pleasanter drug tamoxifen. Screening has been accompanied by a much greater use of breast-conserving treatments, but the assumption that loss of the breast was a key factor in causing psychiatric morbidity in breast cancer patients has been challenged. Dean et al. [5] in a trial in which patients were randomly allocated to a group having immediate breast reconstruction or a group offered it a year later found that it was only among patients with marital problems and those for whom body image was particularly important that postponement of breast reconstruction made a difference to psychosexual and social morbidity. Fallowfield et al. [12] found, among patients who had given informed consent to be randomised, that those allocated to mastectomy were no more distressed than those with breast conservation. They concluded that the threat to life was more important than change of body image. Kiebert et al. [21], reviewing 18 studies on mastectomy versus conservation, concluded that there was reasonably consistent evidence of sexual and cosmetic advantage from conservation but no advantage in terms of reduced anxiety and depression. More recent studies [13, 24, 39] similarly failed to demonstrate any reduction in anxiety and depression among patients receiving breast-conserving treatment for early stage cancer. The benefit of a smaller operation may be offset by the greater likelihood that adjuvant radiotherapy will be advised. Among patients randomised to receive radiotherapy Omne-Ponten et al. [39] found more distress during the first three months but less distress later on. Whether this was a radiotherapy-induced effect, a result of having to keep attending hospital or because of varying interpretations of the implications of such treatment is uncertain.

Returning to the question "Is the distress of cancer found by screening more intense, long lasting or different in quality from that of cancers presenting with symptoms?" it must be noted that there has been more speculation than investigation. No difference between screen-detected and symptom-presenting cancer patients was found in the study by Ellman et al. [8] but the sample was small. Haddad and Maguire [17] have started a larger study of the psychological morbidity associated with mode of diagnosis and in a preliminary report of early findings observe slightly, but not significantly, more affective disorder in the symptomatic group rather than in the screen-detected group of cancer patients (21% versus 16%).

Since screening increases, often by many years, the length of Phase 4 the quality of life during this phase is very important to any assessment of the net benefit from screening. Psychological morbidity is still commonly present 12 months after diagnosis though not as prevalent as during the first 3 months [30]. Morris et al. [35], on the basis of a study in which 34 patients were followed for 2 years, concluded that a substantial proportion of patients suffered from permanent sorrow after mastectomy. This was not consistent with findings in a more recent study in which anxiety and depression were compared between cancer patients attending for mammographic screening of their remaining breast, and a comparable sample who had not had breast cancer [10]. The aim was to assess the quality of life of apparently cured patients after their period of initial adjustment. The study covered 76% of all surviving breast cancer patients who were first diagnosed during a seven year Trial of Early Detection of Breast Cancer [50]. The women had survived for 2-13 years since diagnosis and women with active recurrent or metastatic breast cancer were excluded. The scores on the HAD scale were lower among the apparently cured cancer patients than among the control women without breast cancer. Among these cancer patients there was no difference between those whose cancer had been screen-detected and those who had been symptomatic. Hall [18] similarly found that a higher proportion of breast cancer patients reported good health than a "convenience sample" of women of the same age. A possible explanation for the lack of complaint among the now apparently disease-free cancer patients may be that the acute distress of an earlier experience leads to greater tolerance of relatively minor distressful emotions. Several patients state that coming through a distressing experience has given them a better outlook on life but this cannot be objectively balanced against the opposing view [36] that cancer treatment leaves a permanent "silent sadness". In the absence of stronger proof to the contrary, it seems reasonable to accept that the enjoyment of life by patients who have had time to get over the immediate effects of diagnosis and treatment and have a low probability of death from the disease in the next five years is as good as that of other people.

Reducing Distress – Improving Attendance

Minimising distress attributable to screening is desirable both in itself and because it leads to better future attendance at screening. Given that breast and cervical screening programmes when properly organised result in a reduction of mortality and metastatic disease and that the chance of benefit outweighs the chance of harm to those who attend, the main way in which the psychological as well as physical benefits of the programmes can be increased is by ensuring that programmes are well-organised and reach a high proportion of the target population.

Publicity through radio, television, newspapers and posters is helpful in preparing those targeted for a screening programme if they are thereby persuaded that the tests are widely approved and that they are vulnerable to the disease. Publicity may, however, deter some from attending if it exaggerates the risk and unpleasantness of the disease. Among screening volunteers with a family history of cancer greater fear of the disease was related to more erratic compliance with advice [26]. People may be more encouraged by the belief that others expect them to go for screening [51] than by a belief that it will make a very dramatic difference to risk.

Preparation for a screening programme must include adequate information for general practitioners and other health professionals who may be asked by those exhorted to attend screening to endorse the recommendation and answer queries. Personal letters, preferably giving a specific appointment [7], result in the highest attendance rates [49, 55]. The letter should explain the purpose of screening and give practical details of where to go and what to expect. Local consumer opinion should be consulted on the contents, intelligibility and acceptability.

The amount of information which should be given is controversial. The American Cancer Society recommends detailed information and would like all screenees to give written consent beforehand acknowledging that they have been told about the risks of false positives and false negatives [23]. However, the salient facts are not precisely known and can vary from screening programme to programme. How a subject responds depends not simply on the probabilities of harm and benefit but on how they are presented [20]; more people would choose a 98% chance of survival than would make the same choice if presented as a 2% risk of death. Statements about the life-time risk of cancers or of cancer death may give an exaggerated sense of risk by failing to point out that much of the risk is only experienced in extreme old age. An estimate of risk tailored to the subject's age group and family history of cancer and carefully explained, is relevant to those faced with a choice of screening or prophylactic treatment [26].

Several studies of consumer opinion have sought to identify the factors contributing to anxiety. Receipt of the letter may suddenly make people aware of their vulnerability to cancer or make them feel threatened that if they do not comply with advice they will be blamed later for what happens to them. Among non-attenders [29] a general dread of medical encounters or superstitious fear of the mention of cancer may be evoked.

Surveys of women's opinion about breast screening in the UK [8] have found that only a small proportion of those questioned, 9% of those recalled but less than 1% of those passed as screen-negative, were critical but diverse complaints were voiced.

Women were distressed by difficulty in following directions, by delays – especially when unexpected and unexplained – by embarrassment over their partial nudity, or inability to control expression of pain, by thoughtless remarks of staff, by claustrophobia, by fear of contamination from dressing-gowns which others had used.

Complaints of discomfort or pain feature in all consumer surveys on mammographic screening but the prevalence of pain varies. Rutter et al. [44] found that 6% complained of pain and a further 35% of discomfort whereas Stomper et al. [46] reported that only 1% experienced pain and 10% discomfort. The difference might be due to differences in the pressure applied. Complaint about the discomfort of mammography was sometimes associated with fears that bruising is a cause of breast cancer, that radiation may cause breast cancer or that compression may cause dissemination of cancer cells, suggesting a need to reassure some people that pain is not a sign of serious damage.

Surveys of consumer opinion may indicate which problems are locally most important. Factors affecting attendance can be grouped into simple obstacles such as inaccessibility and ignorance and psychological factors such as attitudes to risk taking and prevention, fear of medical interventions, beliefs about personal vulnerability and the behaviour approved by relatives and friends. The psychological factors are more difficult to alter.

Most studies have been on women attending screening for the first time but have included a question on intention to come again. Orton et al. [40] confirmed, by questioning attenders and non-attenders of later screening rounds, that it is those who are more critical – of the attitude of staff, of discomfort during mammography and of delays – who fail to return. These are aspects of screening which can be improved, though possibly at some extra cost, but it is difficult to know to what extent attendance would be improved by changing physical circumstances. Criticisms may be offered to justify attitudes to reattendance where the real reasons are more difficult to express. Even where delays are not shortened and the method of screening unchanged, prior warning and assurance that the process is harmless may reduce distress and hence improve future compliance.

Reduction in the Distress Caused by Recall

Even though the majority of people asked to compare the stress of recall with other common experiences rate it as minor [14], the stress should be minimised by limiting the number recalled and shortening the period during which the subject is left in suspense. Both the shock of recall and the distress of waiting may to some extent be reduced by forewarning but anxious patients often admit that they have overlooked the information given in a letter. More explanation must accompany the recall letter and it is helpful to give a phone number of someone who can answer urgently any worrying questions.

Follow-up investigation should be provided by specialist screening teams who can provide optimal management and attention to those details which help to reduce distress. Training should be given to the staff in recognising severe anxiety and depression, eliciting the particular causes of it in individual patients and in giving accurate information in the least alarming way possible. It is helpful for patients to have the opportunity to come back with more questions after their first attempt at digesting bad news and hence a nurse counsellor who knows what a patient has been told and can explain the implications is particularly helpful at recall clinics. It is also essential that GPs, who may be asked for advice by the patient, should be promptly informed about the situation.

The distress of a false positive screen is much dependent on whether further investigation entails surgical biopsy [14] or laparotomy [53]. Overtreatment, defined here as meaning treatment for conditions which would not have progressed to invasive cancer even if left unnoticed, gets much less mention than underdiagnosis because it is usually difficult to prove in individual cases. Attempts to quantify the extent of overtreatment of cervical neoplasia using epidemiological evidence [16, 52] suggest that more than half the women treated under the age of 35 years would never have developed the disease. Overdiagnosis of neuroblastoma is also suspected where mass screening yields detection rates higher than the expected cumulative lifetime incidence (Chapter 8). This is also the case in prostate cancer (Chapter 7).

Staff Stress

The necessity of controlling the cost of screening by maximising throughput often gives the screener little time in which to explain procedures and convince patients of her/his sympathy. The screener has also to deal with the annoyance and anxiety caused by the occasional hitch in services. It is not surprising, therefore, that almost a third of British radiographers providing mammographic screening report that they find their work stressful [27]. Screening may also elicit anxiety in staff because of fear of making a wrong judgement, missing a cancer or simply having to deal with upset patients. Valid causes for criticism of staff can be reduced through good organisation and training. There is a temptation to take other actions which might theoretically reduce the chance of missing a cancer and so reduce staff anxiety, such as reducing throughput, shortening the interval between screens, introducing more double checks, lowering the threshold for recalling patients or recommending surgical investigations. Before such steps are taken full consideration must be given to whether the action is merely defensive or is in the best interests of screenees and of the whole eligible population. Stress among staff may also be reduced by ensuring a supportive staff structure in which regular meetings permit discussion of problems and sharing of responsibility. Regular testing to prove competence may help to protect staff against the anxiety that a single decision which, with hindsight, appeared mistaken might unfairly lead to censure.

Surveys of user satisfaction are helpful to staff in that complaints can be put into context. It is usually only a small minority of attenders who are dissatisfied and appreciative comments improve morale, leading to a better response to justifiable criticisms.

Self-Screening

An alternative to screening by professionals is screening by the subjects themselves. This has been advocated as a regular monthly activity for breast cancer and, less frequently, for melanoma. There is no strong evidence that regular self-screening is effective but this may be because it is difficult to mount suitable trials [9]. The desire to "do something", even though there is no evidence that prevention of metastatic disease is possible through early detection, leads frequently to the suggestion that self-examination should be practised.

There are three necessary conditions for success from self-examination. The subjects must carry out the examinations at sufficiently frequent intervals, they must be able to recognise significant changes and distinguish them from non-significant ones, and they must refer themselves promptly to an expert in early diagnosis if signs are found.

In a study of breast self-examination (BSE) conducted by Huguley and Brown [19] it was found that some patients said they had found their cancers by self-examination and yet 9% delayed more than 6 months before they consulted anyone. Health education alone is not enough to promote early action; easy access to professionals whom the patient trusts is equally important.

In a breast screening programme where women were receiving annual professional screeeening, staff encouraged BSE or breast awareness provided it did not cause anxiety. Comments by women showed that some with nodular breasts feared to be considered neurotic if they presented every time a new breast lump was discovered, and found it difficult to remember what had been felt last month. If self-examination was practised in the evening worry could cause loss of sleep. There was no evidence of obsessional self-examination [8].

For melanoma, campaigns have been organised in which the public are encouraged to examine their skin moles. The problem with these is that they produce a sudden flood of worried patients and consequent delays within the dermatology services (Chapter 5).

Selective Screening

This chapter has been concerned chiefly with mass screening in which the only selection for invitation is on the basis of age and sex. Screening for high risk groups identified by genetic, environmental or behavioural factors may present special psychological difficulties. Screening for those at high familial risk is recommended for a small number of rare cancers, e.g. medullary thyroid cancer and retinoblastoma. For most common cancers, however, it has not been widely encouraged. This may change as defective genes are precisely identified making it possible to distinguish carriers who may have a more than 80% chance of developing cancer from non-carriers. As with other forms of genetic screening counselling will be needed before such screening to inform individuals about the test accuracy and discuss whether the prophylaxis or close surveillance to which a positive screen would lead would be acceptable. Judging from experience with screening for Huntington's chorea, non-carriers in high risk families are not necessarily relieved on hearing the test outcome [47].

Selective screening for men exposed to bladder carcinogens at work and women at risk from chorioncarcinoma following a trophoblastic disease pregnancy are accepted practices which have not attracted much attention from psychologists.

It has sometimes been suggested that screening for common cancers should be better targeted on those at highest risk (e.g. for cervical cancer, poor women or women with more sex partners; for breast cancer, those who had no children before age 30 years), or that special approaches should be made to those who are less compliant (e.g. immigrants). The likelihood of greater cost-effectiveness or improved attendance must be balanced against the risk of adding to distress among those who may already feel frightened of cancer or stigma.

Conclusions and Further Research Needs

Attempts to quantify the distress attributable to screening have tended to modify views about the extent of the distress, indicating that it is short-lived and manageable, a reasonable price to pay. Thus, where the sensitivity and specificity of screening are high and the value of early diagnosis in saving lives and reducing morbidity are not in doubt, psychological benefit is likely to accompany physical benefit. Conflicting messages about the value of a screening programme, on the other hand, contribute to anxiety.

There is a continuing need for review of practice and consumer opinion to ensure that unnecessary causes of distress are minimised but large, controlled trials of the psychological effects of screening are difficult to conduct and unless very well conducted may simply reinforce prejudices or be ignored.

References

1. Brandberg Y, Bolund C, Michelson H, Mansson-Brahme E, Ringborg U, Sjoden P-O (1993) Psychological reactions in public melanoma screening. Eur J Cancer 29A(6):860–863.
2. Bull AR, Campbell MJ (1991) Assessment of the psychological impact of a breast screening programme. Br J Radiol 64:510–515.
3. Campion MJ, Brown JR, McCance DJ, Atia W et al. (1988) Psychosexual trauma of an abnormal cervical smear. Br J Obstet Gynaecol 95:175–181.
4. Cockburn J, Staples M, Hurley SF, de Luise T (1994) Psychological consequences of screening mammography. J Med Screening 1:7–12.
5. Dean C, Chetty U, Forrest APM (1983) Effects of immediate breast reconstruction on psychosocial morbidity after mastectomy. Lancet i:459–462.
6. Dean C, Roberts MM, French K, Robinson S (1986) Psychiatric morbidity after screening for breast cancer. J Epidemiol Community Health 40:71–75.

7. Eardley A, Elkind A (1990) A pilot study of attendance for breast cancer screening. Soc Sci Med 30(6):693–699.
8. Ellman R, Angeli N, Christians A, Moss S, Chamberlain J, Maguire P (1989) Psychiatric morbidity associated with screening for breast cancer. Br J Cancer 60:781–784.
9. Ellman R, Moss S, Coleman D, Chamberlain J (1993) Breast self-examination programmes in the trial of early detection of breast cancer: ten year findings. Br J Cancer 68:208–212.
10. Ellman R, Thomas BA (1995). Psychological well-being is not impaired in long-term survivors of breast cancer. J Med Screening 2:5–9
11. Eng C, Stratton M, Ponder B et al. (1994) Familial cancer syndromes. Lancet 343:709–713.
12. Fallowfield LJ, Baum M, Maguire GP (1986) Effects of breast conservation on psychological morbidity associated with diagnosis and treatment of early breast cancer. Br Med J 293:1331–1334.
13. Goldberg JA, Scott RN, Davidson PM, Murray GD et al. (1992) Psychological morbidity in the first year after breast surgery. Eur J Surg Oncol 18(4):327–331.
14. Gram IT, Lund R, Slenker SE (1990) Quality of life following a false positive mammogram. Br J Cancer 62:1018–1022.
15. Gram IT, Slenker SE (1992) Cancer anxiety and attitudes toward mammography among screening attenders, nonattenders, and women never invited. Am J Public Health 82(2):249–251.
16. Gustafsson L, Adami H-O (1989) Natural history of cervical neoplasia: consistent results obtained by an identification technique. Br J Cancer 60:132–141.
17. Haddad P, Maguire P (1993) Psychiatric morbidity associated with mode of diagnosis. In: Austoker J, Patnick J (eds) Breast screening acceptability: research and practice. NHSBSP Publication No. 28, Sheffield, Trent RHA, p 87.
18. Hall J (1992) A cost-effectiveness analysis of mammography screening in Australia. Soc Sci Med 34(9):993–1004.
19. Huguley CM, Brown RL (1981) The value of breast self-examination. Cancer 47:989–995.
20. Kahneman D, Tversky A (1982) The psychology of preferences. Sci Am 246:136–142
21. Kiebert GM, de Haes JCJM, van de Velde CJH (1991) Impact of breast-conserving treatment and mastectomy on quality of life of early-stage breast cancer patients: a review. J Clin Oncol 9:1059–1070.
22. Kincey J, Statham S, McFarlane T. (1991) Women undergoing colposcopy: their satisfaction with communication, health knowledge and level of anxiety. Health Educ J 50:70–72.
23. Lee JM (1993) Screening and informed consent. N Engl J Med 328:438–439.
24. Lee MS, Love SB, Mitchell JB et al. (1992) Mastectomy or conservation for early breast cancer: psychological morbidity. Eur J Cancer 28A(8/9):1340–1344.
25. Lerman C, Trock B, Rimer BA, Boyce A, Jepson C, Engstrom PF (1991) Psychological and behavioral implications of abnormal mammograms. Ann Intern Med 114:657–661.
26. Lerman C, Schwartz M (1993) Adherence and psychological adjustment among women at high risk for breast cancer. Breast Cancer Res Treat 28:145–155.
27. Lovegrove MJ (1991) What relevance, if any, has health education for the radiographers employed in the Breast Screening Service? Msc Thesis, King's College, University of London.
28. Luesley D (1992) Complications of cone biopsy. Br J Obstet Gynaecol 92:153–164.

29. Maclean U, Sinfield D, Klein S, Harden B (1984) Who declines breast screening? J Epidemiol Community Health 38:278–283.
30. Maguire GP, Lee EG, Bevington DJ, Kuchemann CS, Crabtree RJ, Cornell CE (1978) Psychiatric problems in the first year after mastectomy. Br Med J 1:963–965.
31. Maguire P, van Dam F (1983) Psychological aspects of breast cancer; workshop report. Eur J Cancer 19(12):1735–1740.
32. Maguire P, Selby P (1989) Assessing quality of life in cancer patients. Br J Cancer 60:437–440.
33. Mant D, Fitzpatrick R, Hogg A et al. (1990) Experiences of patients with false positive results from colorectal cancer screening. Br J Gen Pract 40:423–425.
34. Marteau TM (1989) Psychological costs of screening. Br Med J 299:527.
35. Morris T, Greer HS, White P (1977) Psychological and social adjustment to mastectomy. A two-year follow-up study. Cancer 40:2381–2387.
36. Morris T (1987) Silent sadness of the "cured" breast cancer patient. In: Aaronson N, Beckman J (eds) Quality of life of cancer patients. Raven Press, New York, pp 201–206.
37. Nathoo V (1988) Investigation of non-responders at a cervical cancer screening clinic in Manchester. Br Med J 296:1041–1042.
38. National Health Service Breast Screening Programme (1993) Breast screening acceptability: research and practice. Austoker J, Patnick J (eds) NHSBSP Publication No. 28, Trent RHA, Sheffield.
39. Omne-Ponten M, Holmberg L, Burns T, Adami HO, Bergstrom R (1992) Determinants of the psycho-social outcome after operation for breast cancer. Results of a prospective comparative interview study following mastectomy and breast conservation. Eur J Cancer 28A(6/7):1062–1067.
40. Orton M, Fitzpatrick R, Fuller A, Mant D, Mlynek C, Thorogood M (1991) Factors affecting women's response to an invitation to attend for a second breast screening examination. Br J Gen Pract 1:303–313.
41. Posner T, Vessey M (1988) Prevention of cervical cancer. The patient's view. King Edward's Hospital Fund for London, London.
42. Reelick NF, de Haes WF, Schuurman JII (1984) Psychological side-effects of the mass screening of cervical cancer. Soc Sci Med 18:1089–1093.
43. Roberts MM (1989). Breast screening: time for a re-think. Br Med J 229:1153–1155.
44. Rutter DR, Calnan M, Vaile MSB, Field S, Wade KA (1992) Discomfort and pain during mammography: description, prediction and prevention. Br Med J 305:443–445.
45. Sprangers MAG, Aaronson KA (1992) The role of health care providers and significant others in evaluating the quality of life of patients with chronic disease: a review. J Clin Epidemiol 45:743–760.
46. Stomper PC, Kopans DB, Sadowsky NL et al. (1988) Is mammography painful? A multicentre patient survey. Arch Intern Med 148:521–524.
47. Tibben A (1993) What is knowledge but grieving? On psychological effects of presymptomatic DNA testing for Huntington's disease. PhD Thesis, Rotterdam.
48. Torrance GW (1986) Measurement of health state utilities for economic appraisal: a review. J Health Econ 5:1–30.
49. Turnbull D, Irwig L, Adelson P (1991) A randomised trial of invitations to attend for screening. Aust J Public Health 15:33–36.
50. UK Trial of Early Detection of Breast Cancer Group (1988) First results on mortality reduction in the UK Trial of Early Detection of Breast Cancer. Lancet ii:411–416.
51. Vaile MSB, Calnan M, Rutter DR, Wall B (1993) Breast cancer screening services in three areas: uptake and satisfaction. J Publ Health Med 15(1):37–45.

52. van Oortmarssen GJ, Habbema JDF (1991) Epidemiological evidence for age-dependent regression of pre-invasive cervical cancer. Br J Cancer 64:559–565.
53. Wardle FJ, Collins W, Pernet AL, Whitehead MI, Bourne TH, Campbell S (1993) Psychological impact of screening for familial ovarian cancer. J Natl Cancer Inst 85:653–657.
54. Wilkinson C, Jones JM, McBride J (1990) Anxiety caused by abnormal result of cervical smear test: a controlled trial Br Med J 300:440.
55. Wilson A, Leeming A (1987) Cervical cytology: a comparison of two call systems. Br Med J 295:181–182.
56. Wright C (1986) Breast cancer screening: a different look at the evidence. Surgery 100(4):594–598.

10 – Economic Aspects of Cancer Screening
Jackie Brown

Introduction

Recognition that resources are limited has led to a growing concern for efficiency in the provision of health care in the UK, which has been heightened with the advent of the recent NHS reforms. Purchasing agencies, such as fundholding general practitioners, and providers, such as hospital trusts, are now expected to take on the more traditional economic roles of consumers and producers, responding to market mechanisms and improving, in the process, the efficiency of health care delivery [48]. Clinton's health reform plan for the US takes a parallel position, whereby it is proposed that large groups of American employers act as purchasing agencies who will negotiate with insurers. They, in turn, will negotiate with doctors to find high quality care at the lowest cost [42]. It should not be surprising, therefore, to learn that the demand for economic skills has grown alongside these changes. One of the most important sets of skills that economists can offer in this context is that of economic appraisal techniques. These help decision makers (both purchasers and providers) to address three particular questions: which health care programmes are worthwhile undertaking, whether alternative configurations of the programmes, other than the existing ones, result in better value for money and how such programmes should be organised so that scarce resources are not needlessly wasted.

Economic appraisal techniques are thus being increasingly used in health care to aid decisions about alternative courses of actions. In the case of cancer screening, for example, economic appraisal can contribute to decisions about whether to introduce a new screening programme for a particular disease site, such as colorectal cancer, or whether to make changes within existing programmes, such as reducing the interval between screens within the current UK breast screening programme.

The aims of this chapter are 3-fold: to explain the need for economic appraisal; to discuss the available methods for evaluation and to consider under what circumstances it is appropriate to use these techniques. Specific examples are taken from the existing literature on screening and used both to illustrate and clarify issues, and to draw attention to the need to take care when seeking to draw more general conclusions from individual studies.

The Need for Economic Appraisal

Economic appraisal is concerned with assessing the efficiency of the way in which scarce resources are used. Instead of relying on methods such as educated guesses or "gut feelings" to make choices over the deployment of scarce resources (such as people's time, buildings and equipment) a number of analytical techniques have been produced by economists to aid their efficient allocation. Each technique is concerned with systematically comparing both the inputs (or costs) and the outputs (or consequences) of alternative courses of action, but differ in how they measure and value the consequences of such actions [16].

Economic appraisal techniques are a way of organising thinking about, and carrying out measurement of, the consequences identified with alternative courses of action. They are only intended as an aid to decision making, because criteria other than efficiency, such as equity, may also be relevant when judging health care alternatives. Nonetheless economists will argue that economic appraisal should go hand in hand with resource allocation decision making. This belief stems from the economists' premise that resources are scarce and that a choice to implement one particular health care programme necessarily uses resources which have an "opportunity cost" in terms of the benefits that could have been derived had the resources been deployed to the alternative programme(s) available.

Prices act as signals to producers in the competitive market. High prices, for example, reflect scarcity of supply relative to consumers' demands and act as an incentive to suppliers to direct resources into the production of goods or services best suited to satisfying consumers' desires. In the public sector, however, such signals tend not to exist, as products are usually "free" at the point of consumption. In the UK, for example, prior to the introduction of the recent reforms, the health care market was provider driven. It still remains to be seen how effectively the purchasing agencies and providers will take on the roles of consumers and producers, following the reforms, and mimic a more competitive market.

Methods for Economic Evaluation

There are several economic appraisal methods available, the appropriateness of which will depend on the nature of the question being addressed. In principle, the most comprehensive of these techniques is cost–benefit analysis which accepts the proposition that an efficient allocation of resources is necessary to maximise the economic welfare of society. The criterion of efficiency is based on a comparison of the value placed on the outputs of a programme, or intervention, with that placed on the required inputs. Thus an efficient programme is one whereby the benefits exceed the costs. Where there are multiple alternatives under comparison, the implication is that one with the greatest benefit, net of costs, should be implemented. This technique necessarily implies that the programme's outputs and resource costs are measured in the same unit of account, i.e. money. Contrary to the claim often made in the titles of some studies, however, in practice true cost–benefit analyses are rarely undertaken to evaluate health care programmes because of the difficulties associated with valuing health outcomes in monetary terms.

Cost-effectiveness analysis attempts to overcome this problem by defining the benefit or "effectiveness" of a health care programme in terms of natural units, such as life-years gained, cases cured or cases of disease detected. No attempt is made to value outcome. Indeed where the outcomes of two programmes are the same, or similar, cost-minimisation is all that is necessary whereby only the resource uses of alternatives are compared [43]. Results of a cost-effectiveness analysis are presented in terms of a cost-effectiveness ratio, such as the cost per case detected, the implication being that those programmes capable of generating a given output for the least cost, or the most output for a given a cost, are implemented. This type of analysis is useful for determining "technical efficiency", i.e. the most efficient way of delivering a particular programme, such as which test to use in a screening programme. It may also be useful for comparing alternative programmes whose effects can be measured in the same units. It is not, however, very helpful if effectiveness is measured in different units. Nor is it of any use to evaluate a single programme, since there is nothing to compare the cost-effectiveness ratio with, nor is it very helpful if programmes have several clinical effects such as changes in morbidity and mortality [51].

Cost–utility analysis, however, attempts to measure the health effects of all programmes in a generic unit. It may be considered a special case of cost-effectiveness analysis whereby the value of a programme's effects are measured in terms of utility. Utility reflects the preferences of individuals or society and, in the context of health care appraisal, refers to the value placed on a specific health status or an improvement in health status. The most common measure of utility used in such analyses is the health-related quality-adjusted life-year or QALY. It incorporates both the programme's impact on survival as well as health related quality of life [16]. Where outcomes are multidimensional, QALYs are useful for determining technical efficiency. More controversially, QALYs can also be used to help judge relative priorities across different programmes in health care. Procedures can be ranked according to their marginal (additional) cost per QALY gained and, on the basis of a fixed budget for health care, programmes having the least cost per QALY are given the highest priority. One of the main implications of these rankings, so-called "QALY league tables", however, is that the only output of the health service is health and, thus, that the only foregone outcomes arising from the resource use considered in these tables are health outcomes. This means that resource use from outside the health budget and non-health outcomes are difficult to incorporate into such tables. In addition, reservations have been expressed, for example, with the regards to the quality of data used in such studies, as well as the difficulties of comparing studies undertaken in different years. Analysts have also been criticised for not providing an adequate account of the marginal analysis undertaken. Moreover, individual cost–utility studies are often locally specific as the appropriate comparator for the decision-making context may differ between localities. It may also be inappropriate to transfer results to another area if, for example, the incidence and prevalence of the disease or level of service differs between two areas. Thus caution in using such tables has been recently urged by some economists [17, 23, 36]. Nonetheless, it should be recognised that resource allocation does take place and that QALYs can be used to aid such decisions, but they are in their early stages of development and should be viewed as being indicative rather than determinate.

In addition, cost–utility analysis is not possible if data on the effectiveness of final outcomes is not available. Moreover, it is unnecessary if the programmes under comparison are all equally effective, or quality of life can be captured in easily understood natural units, or the results cannot be altered by the use of utility values [51].

Thus economic appraisal may take a number of forms, depending on the questions being posed and data available. Cost–benefit and, more controversially, cost–utility analysis can be used to determine allocative efficiency. They address the issue of outcome valuation and thus can determine whether a particular health care programme is "worthwhile" when compared to other health care programmes. The fact that a programme is worthwhile is, however, an inherent assumption in cost-effectiveness analysis which is more appropriate for determining the most efficient way of delivering a particular programme or treatment for a particular condition.

Economic Appraisal of Cancer Screening Programmes

The UK national breast screening programme was introduced following the recommendations of the Forrest report [21]. The recommendations were made after considering the evidence from overseas randomised trials and the UK trial of the early detection of breast cancer, as well as the results of an economic appraisal. Screening for cervical cancer, on the other hand, was introduced on an *ad hoc* basis and it is unlikely that economic appraisal can now influence whether screening will continue, given the support of both the government and medical profession for the programme. Economic appraisal can, however, influence changes within such programmes, such as whether the age of screening should be reduced or the frequency of screening increased.

Moreover, economic appraisal can influence the introduction of new cancer screening programmes such as those recently proposed for colorectal [9, 28], prostate [8, 47], ovarian [2, 29] and oral cancers [20, 38]. Here the analyst is interested in the resulting change in costs and outcomes compared to the scenario of no formal organised screening; whereas the evaluation of changes to an existing screening programme involves estimating the difference in costs and outcomes relative to the existing screening programme, i.e. it is the incremental (or marginal) costs and outcomes of expansion, or contraction, of a programme which are relevant not the total costs and total outcomes of the programme.

The Outcomes of a Screening Programme

The outcomes used in economic evaluation can only be as good as the clinical evidence upon which they are based. Ideally, this evidence should come from population-based prospective randomised controlled trials. In the case of cancer screening the main measure would obviously be reduced mortality, but other attributes may well be relevant. For example, there is general agreement that screening may also affect the screenee's health-related quality of life. For individuals with cancer (or premalignant disease) true positive screening results will bring forward the time of detection. The resulting health-related quality of life experienced between detection and death thus needs to be compared with that experienced when no organised screening takes place. In addition, a number of health states are likely to be experienced between detection and death. Moreover, different patients will not necessarily experience the same ones. Nonetheless one might expect earlier detection to reduce the severity of illness experienced and hence improve quality of life. False negative screening results, on the other hand, may delay diagnosis and lead to the development of more advanced cancer.

Evidence also exists from breast and cervical screening programmes to suggest that psychiatric morbidity is, at least temporarily, raised by attendance for screening and follow-up assessment examinations, especially for women who have false positive results [7, 19, 24, 35]. Other work suggests that psychiatric morbidity may also be experienced by non-attenders [34].

In addition, non-health related effects, such as reassurance from a negative test, and other information which does not affect prognosis or subsequent treatment, may be gained through screening [6, 26]. Non-health effects such as pain and discomfort caused by the test itself, for example that caused by mammography, may also be an important outcome [25].

Thus all possible outcomes of a screening programme, i.e. those incurred by individuals who have either true positive, false positive, false negative, or true negative results and the non-attenders needs to be compared with those outcomes which would otherwise occur if no organised screening were to take place [49].

QALYs are one way of incorporating health-related quality of life into an economic appraisal, but while going a long way to incorporating quality of life considerations into the outcome measure, to date the application of the quality-adjusted life year approach has not succeeded in incorporating non-health benefits such as reassurance. In order to estimate QALYs, different health states are not just ranked but weights are attached to them. Thus value judgements are made as to the relative importance of avoiding one state compared to another. Health states are valued on a cardinal scale, of the ratio type, which enables one to say not only that the interval between numbers is the same but also that health state 6 is three times as bad as health state 2.

There is, however, disagreement as to how such ill health states should be evaluated. One approach is to use a multiattribute scale of health state utilities. Any health state is disaggregated into its component dimensions, such as physical functioning and mental state, and scores are assigned to each dimension. Each score is then assigned a predetermined weight and incorporated into an overall scale [27]. These generalised methods, however, have been criticised as being too insensitive to some aspects of quality of life [32], although they do allow comparisons to be made across health care programmes.

As an alternative, health state descriptions can be developed which are specific to the disease or condition under consideration. Whether the generalised multiattribute scale or disease specific valuations are used, the estimation of QALYs usually involves deriving the weights for a series of health states and then applying them to the years spent in that health state. Weights are usually assigned on a scale from one to zero, where zero is worst imaginable health and one is best imaginable health [39, 51].

There is some evidence to suggest that values may be influenced, among other things, by the duration of the health condition and the expected prognosis. Thus Hall [27] used the Healthy Year Equivalents approach whereby scenarios of health states over time are presented to individuals for valuation. Another methodological issue arises over whose values should be used for the specific health states or scenarios, for example, in order to value health states associated with breast cancer screening de Haes et al. [13] used the values of 12 "experts" in breast cancer and 15 employees of the Department of Public Health and Social Medicine. Buxton et al. [4] used a sample of hospital doctors, general practitioners, nurses and general university staff and Hall [27] used the values of 104 women with and without breast cancer in the age group relevant for screening.

The most common techniques used by analysts to value such health states include: standard gamble, the rating scale and time trade-off methods [16, 39, 51]. Each measures slightly different things, but Mooney and Olsen [37] have argued that the time trade-off method serves the purpose most appropriately as it addresses choices in the context of trading off quantity and quality of life, choices most closely related to the resource allocation decision. The method has been used in the literature to value health states associated with breast cancer [4, 27, 45].

Adjusting the outcome measure for quality of life effects, however, was found to have relatively little effect on the overall estimate of the cost-effectiveness ratio presented in the Forrest report [21]. The Rosser index [44] used to adjust for quality in that analysis is, however, a general quality of life index which is likely to be insensitive to important cancer/breast cancer effects, such as living with a diagnosis of cancer, fear of recurrence, assumed independent of time. Moreover, no account was made of the fact that screening brought forward the time of diagnosis nor was the reduction in health-related quality of life arising from false screening results considered.

A Dutch study [13] while using disease specific measures also found the quality effects inconsequential; however, the interview used to elicit the values of different health states was complicated and the sample size small. Furthermore, the outcomes described were independent of time.

As outlined earlier a different approach was taken in the study by Hall [27] who found that the quality of life adjustments more than doubled the cost-effectiveness ratio. In this Australian study healthy life-year equivalents were estimated rather than quality-adjusted life-years and it was suggested that the utility scale used in the Forrest report was insensitive to the health states associated with breast cancer. Buxton et al. [4] also used disease specific health states and obtained values very different from those obtained by the Rosser index.

Nonetheless, as previously highlighted, all these measures fail to include all the quality of life effects. It therefore remains debatable as to whether quality of life associated with breast cancer has an important effect on the results of these types of economic appraisal. Clearly more research is needed.

Cervical screening, on the other hand, was introduced without any clinical trials being undertaken. Economic studies evaluating cervical screening are nonetheless found in the literature. Most measure effectiveness in terms of lives or life-years gained with no adjustment for quality of life [3], but the evidence of effectiveness is obviously based on more limited epidemiological data. Thus assumptions regarding the effectiveness of cervical screening are likely to differ between studies and this needs to be appreciated when interpreting results and drawing conclusions from such studies. To overcome the lack of data some authors have used computer simulation to model the natural history of the disease and the effects of different screening policies. One of the most recent examples uses a model based on data collected from a Dutch pilot study of organised screening [31].

Although a randomised controlled trial to show the effectiveness of cervical screening would now be impossible to organise as both women and the medical profession now believe in the effectiveness of cervical screening, such trials could be used to determine the outcomes of different referral policies for women with mildly dyskaryotic smears or the outcomes of alternative management strategies of women referred for colposcopy [3].

Where mortality data have not been available, other studies have measured effectiveness in terms of the number of cancers detected. For example, Walker et al. [54] compared the cost-effectiveness of possible screening strategies for colorectal cancer in terms of the additional cost per case detected. It is, however, difficult, if not impossible, to infer the benefit from the number of cases detected. Increased survival does not necessarily follow detection. Moreover, the results of these studies may be misleading as they exclude other important health outcomes such as the impact of quality of life, not only for true positive cases, but for all those screened.

The Costs of a Screening Programme

The costs relevant to appraisal are those incurred and those avoided as a result of undertaking a particular programme. Moreover, it is the opportunity cost, i.e. the value of the outputs that the resources could be redirected to produce, which the economist seeks to estimate for comparison with the programme's benefits. When estimating the costs of introducing or expanding a programme one needs to be clear about the size and nature of the change as it is the marginal rather than average cost which is of interest to the analyst. For example when a service is operating below capacity, the incremental cost of screening an extra individual is likely to be less than the average cost per screen since average costs are likely to include an element of overheads which will not increase as the number screened increases.

Inevitably it will be the direct costs, i.e. those associated with organising and operating the screening programme, such as labour, overheads and capital, which will be the most important to the health service. In the case of a cervical screening programme, for example, this would include the costs associated with recruiting women to the programme; taking and reading the smears; and the cost related to the diagnosis and treatment of those cases detected offset by the reduction in health service cost associated with less patients requiring a diagnosis and radical treatment at a late stage of the disease. The cost savings associated with reducing the scale of advanced treatment is often given as an argument in favour of screening. In the literature, however, studies estimating the costs of a cervical screening programme have found the health service cost associated with the screen itself to be the largest cost component of the programme. By comparison, the savings in terminal treatment are found to be relatively small [31, 46]. In a detailed study by van Ballegooijen et al. [53], for example, the potential savings to the health service due to the reduction in advanced disease and mortality, as a result of a mass cervical screening programme in the Netherlands, were estimated to amount to only 10% of the cost of a screening programme.

Direct costs may also be borne by the patients and their families. They may, for example, incur out-of-pocket expenses such as travel and childminding costs to attend for screening. In addition, patients and their companions will forego time in order to participate in the health care programme; the opportunity cost of which may be, for example, foregone earnings, leisure or housework. These costs are likely to have an important effect on behaviour, particularly attendance rates. Such costs therefore need to be considered carefully, even if it is not appropriate to include patients costs in the ranking of programmes in "QALY league tables" where the objective can only be to maximise health gains for a fixed health service budget [23].

The analysis of such costs to aid the understanding of behaviour factors is, however, something quite different from the controversial use of earnings data as a measure of the value placed on the outcome of health care programmes. Caution is needed when considering the inclusion of such indirect costs since, among other things, it raises distribution issues. For example, it favours screening programmes in an active male labour force since men are, on average, higher income earners.

Dealing with Uncertainty and Time Preference

Inevitably estimation of the costs and benefits is going to be subject to uncertainty which may affect the overall findings. Thus sensitivity analysis is a technique used by economists to test the robustness of the results by varying the values taken by key parameters [15]. In some studies, however, such an analysis is noticeably absent [3].

One further refinement of economic appraisal takes account of the fact that different health care programmes have different patterns of costs and benefits occurring over a period of time. In the case of a screening programme, for example, the costs will invariably occur before the outcomes. Individuals and society, however, demonstrate what economists call "positive time preference". That is, individuals and society prefer to have finances, or resources, now as opposed to later since they can benefit from them in the mean time. The existence of time preference is evidenced by the existence of interest rates paid on money saved, i.e. we prefer to have money today rather than later. Hence future costs and benefits are "discounted", or reduced, to reflect the fact that the costs and benefits occurring in the future do not count for the same value as those occurring now. Health care programmes are thus evaluated using a systematic assessment of present values of their costs and outcomes. In the UK, the current discount rate for the public sector has been set to 6% per annum, by the Treasury. This rate is thus used in most economic evaluations of health care procedures and is applied consistently over succeeding years of the life of a programme.

Parsonage and Neuburger [40] have, however, examined, among other things, the sources of time preference and argued that in practice it is generally inappropriate to discount non-monetary health benefits; but more evidence is needed [5]. This has very significant implications for the cost-effectiveness of screening programmes, the benefits of which tend to extend many years into the future, since benefits left undiscounted will immediately improve cost-effectiveness ratios.

Some Empirical Findings of Economic Evaluations of Cancer Screening

The literature on cancer screening suggests that programmes are generally not cost saving, but compare favourably in terms of cost-effectiveness with expenditure on some other health care services. In the case of breast screening, for example, the Forrest report [21] estimated a cost per QALY of £3309 for a programme screening women, aged between 50 and 64 years, every three years by single-view mammography. This was argued to be similar to other health service activities currently undertaken, falling somewhere between kidney and heart transplant costs per QALY. However, a screening model using Dutch data [14] produced a lower cost per QALY estimate. Fraser and Clarke [22] point out that this is due to the fact that benefits were estimated over a longer period of time in the Dutch study, with savings in advanced disease, and with a higher attendance rate for screening.

Cervical screening is also often judged to be cost-effective in the literature. For example, a Dutch study [31] estimated the cost per life year saved for various cervical screening policies. The most efficient policy of seven invitations in a woman's lifetime was found to be less cost-effective than a breast screening programme with ten invitations, but was argued to be comparable with other health service expenditures. Similarly, Bethwaite et al. [1] considered various screening policies for New Zealand and argued the cost per life saved through cervical screening every three years to be reasonable when compared to the implicit valuations placed on life for other policies. Caution is, however, required when reaching such conclusions as the majority of studies evaluating cervical screening do not include the quality of life effects [3]. Moreover, such estimates cannot tell us whether screening itself is worthwhile as no valuation is made of the outcomes. In addition, where other studies have used proxies such as the number of smear tests [30, 52] or only include the cost of a smear test [11, 18, 50] comparison with other health care programmes requires caution.

A few other studies have looked at the cost-effectiveness of screening programmes for other cancer sites. For example, Cristofolini et al. [12], after estimating a cost of $400 per year of life saved, recommended a programme for the early detection of melanoma in Italy. No adjustment was made for the quality of life effects which makes comparisons with other health care programmes difficult. Moreover, the difference in cost between early and late treatment was not included.

Estimates are also presented in the literature, on the cost-effectiveness of screening for prostate cancer. Chodak [10] and Pederson [41], for example, claim that the cost per case detected by a single digital rectal examination is less than that associated with other screening programmes such as those for breast or cervical screening. In an American study Love et al. [33] estimated the cost per life saved due to a prostate screening programme, starting at age 60 years and taking place at intervals of one to five years, to be between $2276 and $3687. The authors also argue that this is favourable compared to other health care programmes. Again these estimates cannot tell us whether screening is worthwhile since no value is given for the health effects and the costs were not compared to the scenario of no organised screening.

Conclusions

It is widely accepted that resources for health care are limited and economic appraisal is playing a more important role where priority setting must inevitably take place and where efficiency is a growing concern. Techniques are available to assess whether the introduction of a new cancer screening programme or changes within an existing programme are worthwhile, but caution is needed when drawing general conclusions from such studies. The inclusion of costs and outcomes may vary between studies as well as the underlying assumptions based on clinical data. It is important to understand what questions are being addressed and realise that an economic analysis can only ever be as good as the data on which is based. Nonetheless, even though economic appraisal may not give the definitive answer for decisions in policy making, it does provide a very useful way of organising thinking about, and carrying out the measurement of, consequences identified with alternative courses of action. Moreover, it should also be emphasised that economic appraisal techniques are ever improving.

Acknowledgements

The author would like to thank Professor Martin Buxton and Karen Gerard for their helpful comments on an earlier draft of this chapter.

References

1. Bethwaite J, Rayner T, Bethwaite P (1986) Economic aspects of screening for cervical cancer in New Zealand. NZ Med J 99:747–751.
2. Bourne TH, Campbell S, Reynolds KM et al. (1993) Screening for early familial ovarian cancer with transvaginal ultrasonography and colour blood flow imaging. Br Med J 306:1025–1029.
3. Brown J, Sculpher M (1993) Economics of screening programmes to prevent cervical cancer. Contemp Rev Obstet Gynaecol 5:221–229.
4. Buxton M, Ashby J, O'Hanlon M (1987) Alternative methods of valuing health states. HERG Discussion Paper No. 2. Health Economics Research Group, Brunel University.
5. Cairns J (1992) Discounting and health benefits: another perspective. Health Econ 1:76–79.
6. Cairns J, Shackley P (1993) Sometimes sensitive, seldom specific: a review of the economics of screening. Health Econ 2:43–53.
7. Campion MJ, Brown JR, McCance DJ et al. (1988) Psychosexual trauma of an abnormal cervical smear. Br J Obstet Gynaecol 95:175–181.
8. Chadwick DJ, Kemple T, Astley JP et al. (1991) Pilot study of screening for prostate cancer in general practice. Lancet 338:613–616.
9. Chamberlain J (1990) Is screening for colorectal cancer worthwhile? Br J Cancer 62:1–3.

10. Chodak GW, Schoenberg HW (1984) Early detection of prostate cancer by routine screening. JAMA 252:3261–3264.
11. Coppleson LW, Brown B (1976) The prevention of carcinoma of the cervix. Am J Obstet Gynecol 125:153–159.
12. Cristofolini M, Bianchi R, Boi S et al. (1993) Analysis of the cost-effectiveness ratio of the health campaign for the early diagnosis of cutaneous melanoma in Trentino, Italy. Cancer 71:370–374.
13. de Haes JCJM, de Koning HJ, van Oortmarssen GJ, van Agt HME, de Bruyn AE, van der Maas PJ (1991) The impact of a breast cancer screening programme on quality-adjusted life-years. Int J Cancer 49:538–544.
14. de Koning HJ, van Ineveld BM, van Oortmarssen GJ et al. (1991) Breast cancer screening and cost-effectiveness; policy alternatives, quality of life considerations and the possible impact of uncertain factors. Int J Cancer 49:531–537.
15. Drummond MF (1989) Principles of economical appraisal in health care. Oxford University Press, Oxford.
16. Drummond MF, Stoddard GL, Torrance GW (1987) Methods for the economic evaluation of health care programmes. Oxford University Press, Oxford.
17. Drummond MF, Torrance G, Mason J (1993) Cost-effectiveness league tables: More harm than good? Soc Sci Med 37:33–40.
18. Eddy DM (1990) Screening for cervical cancer. Ann Internal Med 113:214–226.
19. Ellman R, Angeli N, Christians A, Moss S, Chamberlain J, Maguire P (1989) Psychiatric morbidity associated with screening for breast cancer. Br J Cancer 60:781–784.
20. Feaver GP (1990) Screening for oral cancer and precancer. Dent Pract May, 16–18.
21. Forrest P (1988) Breast Cancer Screening. Report to the Health Minister of England, Wales, Scotland and Northern Ireland. Department of Health and Social Security, HMSO, London.
22. Fraser MN, Clarke PR (1992) Cost-effectiveness of breast cancer screening. The Breast 1:169–172.
23. Gerard K, Mooney G (1993) QALY league tables: handle with care. Health Econ 2:59–64.
24. Gram IT, Lund E, Slenker SE (1990) Quality of life following a false positive mammogram. Br J Cancer 62:1018–1022.
25. Gram IT, Slenker SE (1992) Cancer anxiety and attitudes towards mammography among screening attenders, nonattenders and women never invited. Am J Public Health 82:249–251.
26. Grimes DS (1988) Value of a negative cervical smear. Br Med J 296:1363.
27. Hall J (1992) A cost-utility analysis of mammography screening in Australia. Soc Sci Med 34:993–1004.
28. Hardcastle JD, Chamberlain J, Sheffield J et al. (1989) Randomised controlled trial of faecal occult blood screening for colorectal cancer. Results of the first 107 349 subjects. Lancet i:1160–1164.
29. Jacobs I, Prys Davies A, Bridges J et al. (1993) Prevalence screening for ovarian cancer in post menopausal women by CA 125 measurement and ultrasonography. Br Med J 306:1030–1034.
30. Knox EG (1976) Ages and frequencies for cervical cancer screening. Br J Cancer 34:444–452.
31. Koopmanschap MA, Lubbe KTN, van Oortmarssen GJ, van Agt HMA, van Ballegooijen M, Habbema JDF (1990) Economic aspects of cervical cancer screening. Soc Sci Med 30:1081–1987.

32. Loomes G, McKenzie L (1989) The use of QALYs in health care decision making. Soc Sci Med 28:299–308.
33. Love RR, Fryback DG, Kimbrough SR (1985) A cost-effectiveness analysis of screening for carcinoma of the prostate by digital examination. Med Decis Making 5(3):263–178.
34. MacLean U, Sinfield D, Klein S, Harden B (1984) Women who decline breast screening. J Epidemiol Community Health 38:278–283.
35. Marteau TM, Walker P, Giles J, Smail M (1990) Anxieties in women undergoing colposcopy. Br J Obstet Gynaecol 97:859–861.
36. Mason J, Drummond M, Torrance G (1993) Some guidelines of the use of cost effectiveness league tables. Br Med J 306:570–572.
37. Mooney G, Olsen JA (1991) QALYs: Where next? In: McGuire A, Fenn P, Mayhew K (eds) Providing health care. Oxford University Press, Oxford, pp 120–140.
38. Nally F (1988) Oral cancer (letter). Br Dent J 165:240.
39. Nord E (1992) Methods for quality adjustment of life years. Soc Sci Med 34(5):559–569.
40. Parsonage M, Neuburger H (1992) Discounting health benefits. Health Econ 1:71–76.
41. Pedersen KV, Carlsson P, Varenhorst E, Lofman O, Berglund K (1990) Screening for carcinoma of the prostate by digital rectal examination in a randomly selected population. Br Med J 300:1041–1044.
42. Roberts JC (1993) How Clinton's reforms compare with the NHS. Br Med J 307:820.
43. Robinson R (1993) Cost and cost-minimisation analysis. Br Med J 307:726–728.
44. Rosser R, Kind P (1978) A scale of valuations of states of illness: is there a social consensus? Int J Epidemiol 7:347–358.
45. Sackett DL, Torrence GW (1978) The utility of different health states as perceived by the general public. J Chron Dis 31:697–704.
46. Schneider J, Twiggs LB (1972) The cost of carcinoma of the cervix. Obstet Gynecol 40:851–858.
47. Schroder FH (1993) Prostate cancer: to screen or not to screen? Br Med J 306:407–408.
48. Secretaries of State for Health, Wales, Northern Ireland and Scotland (1989) Working for patients: the health service: caring for the 1990s. HMSO, London.
49. Simpson P, Chamberlain J, Gravelle HSE (1978) Choice of screening tests. J Epidemiol Community Health 32:166–170.
50. Smith A, Chamberlain J (1987) Managing cervical screening. In: Information technology in health care, Issue 4. Kluwer Publishing Ltd, Kingston upon Thames, pp 2–12.
51. Torrance GW (1986) Measurement of health-state utilities for economic appraisal: A review. J Health Econ 5:1–30.
52. van Ballegooijen M, Habbema JDF, van Oortmarssen GJ, Koopmanschap MA, Lubbe JTN, van Agt HME (1992) Preventive pap-smears: balancing costs, risks and benefits. Br J Cancer 65:930–933.
53. van Ballegooijen M, Koopmanschap MA, Tjokrowardojo AJS, van Oortmarssen GJ (1992) Care and costs for advanced cervical cancer. Eur J Cancer 28A:1703–1708.
54. Walker A, Whynes DK, Thomas WM, Chamberlain JO, Hardcastle JD (1991) Retesting positive results in screening for colorectal cancer: a marginal analysis. Appl Econ 23:1015–1017.

Index